MW00711515

Intermittent Fasting

How to Lose Weight, Burn Fat, and Increase Mental Clarity without Having to Give up All Your Favorite Foods

© **Copyright 2018**

All Rights Reserved. No part of this book may be reproduced in any form without permission in writing from the author. Reviewers may quote brief passages in reviews.

Disclaimer: No part of this publication may be reproduced or transmitted in any form or by any means, mechanical or electronic, including photocopying or recording, or by any information storage and retrieval system, or transmitted by email without permission in writing from the publisher.

While all attempts have been made to verify the information provided in this publication, neither the author nor the publisher assumes any responsibility for errors, omissions or contrary interpretations of the subject matter herein.

This book is for entertainment purposes only. The views expressed are those of the author alone, and should not be taken as expert instruction or commands. The reader is responsible for his or her own actions.

Adherence to all applicable laws and regulations, including international, federal, state and local laws governing professional licensing, business practices, advertising and all other aspects of doing business in the US, Canada, UK or any other jurisdiction is the sole responsibility of the purchaser or reader.

Neither the author nor the publisher assumes any responsibility or liability whatsoever on the behalf of the purchaser or reader of these materials. Any perceived slight of any individual or organization is purely unintentional.

Contents

Introduction

With all the different types of dieting plans out there, it can sometimes be difficult to know which one is the best option. Some people like the idea of the ketogenic diet and eating good fats to promote lots of fat loss. Others like to go on a diet plan that helps them lower their blood pressure and reduce their salt intake. Then there are options that are low fat and higher carb, options for cleansing, and so much more. But which one is the best to choose?

This guidebook is going to spend some time looking at intermittent fasting and all the benefits that can come from following this eating plan. Intermittent fasting encourages healthy eating and puts a limit on the processed and junk foods that are common in the American diet. However, more importantly, intermittent fasting focuses on changing the way, and the times, that you eat.

The idea is to allow the body to go on short-term fasts during the week. This can help clean out the body, speed up the metabolism, and naturally help you to cut down on the number of calories that you consume during the week. And since there are different options when it comes to the type of intermittent fast you can go on, you are sure to find a method that works best for you.

This guidebook provides everything you need to know to get started with intermittent fasting. We will explore what intermittent fasting is, how to get started, some of the different methods that go with an intermittent fast, and some of the benefits and side effects that come with this kind of eating plan. Intermittent fasting may be a different way of eating, but it is going to provide you with some amazing benefits.

While the ideas behind fasting are pretty simple to follow, it is a great way to improve almost every aspect of your health. In addition to helping you lose weight and belly fat, an intermittent fast can help you burn fat, fight off some types of cancer, reduce your insulin levels, help keep the mind sharp, fight off and prevent diabetes, and so much more. All it takes is adjusting the times that you eat during the day.

Intermittent fasting has proven to be effective in helping so many people lose weight and feel better. While some of the results are similar to what can be done with continuous calorie restriction, intermittent fasting is often easier to follow than the latter and can even help you maintain more of your lean muscle mass in the process.

Take some time to read through this guidebook and learn everything that you need to know about intermittent fasting!

Chapter 1: What Is Intermittent Fasting?

While there are many different diet plans, one method that is often more effective at helping you work on your health and lose weight is intermittent fasting. This method can do so much for your body, and the ideas behind it are pretty simple.

With intermittent fasting, you need to concentrate on eating healthy and wholesome foods, but there aren't strict requirements on the foods that you eat. With this option, you will focus more on separating your day into two periods, one for eating and one for fasting or abstaining for eating. The second time period, your fasting window, needs to be longer than normal to help you better control your eating habits and the calories that you take in each day to improve your health.

Intermittent fasting and the different methods that go with it have grown in popularity. With all the great health benefits and the relative ease in which people lose weight on this eating plan, it is no wonder that everyone wants to give it a try. Let's take a look at some of the basics that you should know about intermittent fasting before moving on to discuss the benefits, how to get started, and so much more!

The History of Fasting

Fasting is not a new idea. It has been around for thousands of years. Pythagoras extolled the virtues of fasting, St. Catherine of Siena practiced fasting, and Paracelsus, a doctor during the Renaissance period, called fasting a "physician within" all of us. Fasting, in one form or another, is a distinguished tradition, and throughout the centuries, those who follow it claim that fasting can bring spiritual and physical renewal.

In primitive cultures, a fast would be needed before people went to war. It was also considered a coming of age ritual in many cultures. If the people were worried about an angry deity, a fast was often required, and North Americans would do it as a ceremony to avoid issues like famine.

Many of the major religions in the world have implemented fasting as part of their rituals. It can be used as a form of self-control and penitence or enacted for major events within the religion. For example, Judaism has several fasting days each year, including the Day of Atonement and Yom Kippur. In Islam, followers fast during the month of Ramadan. Easter orthodoxy and Roman Catholics will observe a 40-day fast during Lent.

While fasting has been commonly associated with religious and cultural practices in the past, there are times when fasting was used for other things as well. For example, it has often been used as a political protest tool. Mahatma Gandhi and the Suffragettes went under 17 fasts during the struggle for independence for India.

During the 19th century, a practice that is known as therapeutic fasting became popular to prevent illnesses and even treat some when they were done under medical supervision. This became something that grew with the Natural Hygiene Movement and is still popular today. This was seen as a natural way to help clean out the body and prevent illnesses without having to worry so much about taking medicines that could cause many side effects and harm the body.

Today, there are many reasons why someone would choose to go on a fast. They may choose to do it as a part of their religion, to protest something that they are against, or as a way to clean out their bodies and help them lose weight. Fasting has a long history and many different uses, which makes it the perfect choice when you are ready to make some changes in your diet and lifestyle.

The Basics of an Intermittent Fast

Intermittent fasting is less about the foods that you eat – although these can be important – and more about the timing of your meals. With a traditional American diet, you can easily eat nonstop during the day. Many people start with breakfast, have a snack around midmorning, lunch, another snack, a big dinner, and even another snack before bedtime. There are even some healthy eating plans that recommend eating five or six times a day to help you lose weight.

What all these end up doing is allowing us to eat way too many calories during the day. We are feeding the body a constant supply of energy in the form of glucose, but most of it is not being used and is then stored as extra body fat over time. We get into a bad cycle of eating a bunch of carbs and calories, but still wanting more. This cycle is going to cause us to gain weight and a whole host of other health conditions.

With intermittent fasting, you aim to change this cycle. You will learn how to limit your eating windows, not allowing yourself to eat all the time. This can help you reduce how much you take in and can naturally lead to weight loss. There are different options with intermittent fasting. Some ask you to go 24 hours without eating, some ask you to have a few days a week only eating 500 calories, and others ask you to do smaller fasts each day, limiting your eating window to eight hours or so.

No matter which method you choose to go with, you are limiting the amount of time that you can eat during the day. This results in fewer calories, easier weight loss, and more time to enjoy life. Think of all the freedom you will get just by cutting out a few of the meals that you have to plan and make each week!

When you go on an intermittent fast, you will need to consider what diet plan to go on. Many people like the ketogenic diet because it helps increase the fat burning that comes with fasting. However, many other diet plans can work with intermittent fasting as well. Don't try to start without a diet plan. There isn't one diet plan associated with fasting, but if you continue to take in too many calories and cat junk, you are going to have a hard time seeing results on your fast.

There are also different methods that you can choose when it comes to which type of intermittent fast you want. Some people like to go on an alternate day fast. Some like to have a few days a week, and they are really busy anyway when they fast. Others like to have shorter fasts added into each day. All these methods can be effective; you just need to choose the one that fits into your schedule and stick with it.

Do I Need to Worry About Starvation Mode?

One common concern about intermittent fasting is that you will quickly put your body into starvation mode if you try this form of eating. The worry is that these small fasts are going to be enough to ruin the metabolism and make it hard to lose weight or even function properly. The biggest issue here is that this concern is based on the idea that our bodies can't handle any stress, and going even a few hours without food can send it all out of order.

This is not true.

Think back to our ancestors. Did they have a constant stream of food at their disposal? Did they have horrible metabolic effects when they had to go a few days without eating because of famine or because the food was hard to come by? No, their bodies and ours were adapted to handle these shorter times without food to help them, and us, survive.

Starvation mode happens when you go a long time without food. The body starts to recognize that it isn't getting the nutrition that it once did, and so it will slow down the metabolism to keep you alive. However, studies show that it takes 72 hours or more before you start to see this occur. Intermittent fasting usually lasts less than 24 hours in a row. A few go up to 36 hours, but that is all.

These fasts are not going to be long enough even to come close to the body going into starvation mode. Instead, during these short fasts, the body is going to spend time speeding up the metabolism, burning more calories as it goes through your readily available glucose and then moving on to the glycogen stores as well. Since the fast is so short, and with you concentrating on eating wholesome and nutritious foods during your eating windows, your body will burn more calories than normal, and there is no risk of entering starvation mode.

It is important that you stick with the fast that you chose and don't go overboard with this. If you don't eat healthy foods during your eating window, or you choose to eat too few calories during that time, and your fasts are too long, you could risk entering starvation mode and dealing with all the issues that come with that. However, if you follow your chosen intermittent fast well and you eat the right foods, you don't have to worry about this issue.

Who Would Benefit the Most from Intermittent Fasting?

Almost everyone can benefit from going on an intermittent fast. It helps to speed up the metabolism, can give you more energy, puts the body in fat burning mode and often can result in weight loss and health benefits, unlike any other diet plan. People who would benefit the most from starting an intermittent fast are:

- Those who want to lose weight.

- Those who want to change their eating habits.

- Weightlifters and bodybuilders.

- Those who want to learn how to listen to their bodies more and learn when they are hungry, thirsty, or need to deal with something.

- Those who want to make life easier with fewer meals to plan.

- Those who want to improve their heart health.

- Those who want to help fight off diabetes.

- Those who are looking to keep the brain strong and working well.

- Those who are interested in getting rid of belly fat.

Is There Anyone Who Shouldn't Go on an Intermittent Fast?

While an intermittent fast can be a great way to help improve your health and lose weight, some individuals should consider not doing an intermittent fast. These individuals may experience trouble getting the right amount of nutrition through the day when they fast, and they may have to worry about medications or other issues that fasting can aggravate. People who should consider not doing an intermittent fast, or at least should discuss it with their doctor ahead of time, include:

- Children and teenagers who are still developing and growing.

- Women who are currently pregnant.

- Women who are currently breastfeeding.

- People who have recently had surgery and are recovering.

- People with certain eating disorders.

• Those who are currently underweight.

• Those who are dealing with diabetes that is controlled with insulin.

• Some types of medications can be negatively affected by an intermittent fast as well. Make sure to discuss this with your doctor before starting.

Intermittent fasting is a great eating plan that makes it easy for you to lose weight and improve your health. However, concerning the above conditions, it can be a challenge to fast regarding getting adequate nutrition throughout the day, and not just during short eating windows.

Chapter 2: How Does Intermittent Fasting Help Burn Fat and Weight Loss?

When you go on an intermittent fast, you force the body to stop relying on a constant source of glucose to fuel it. Since you go so long without eating, your body still has to look for some form of fuel to help it function and do well. It will resort to burning the stored glycogen of the body, or the stored body fat. Just by doing these short-term fasts each day, you will burn through the extra fat on your body, cut out calories, and lose weight faster than ever before.

Intermittent fasting is all about adding short fasts into your daily life. The goal is to reduce the number of calories that you consume and increase how fast the metabolism runs at the same time. This can result in not only a bunch of great health benefits but also some weight loss as well. But why is intermittent fasting so effective at helping you to burn fat and lose weight? Let's look at some of the ways that intermittent fasting will affect your body and help you get the results that you want.

Intermittent Fasting and How It Affects Your Hormones

The body fat that you carry around is simply just the way that the body stores any unused energy or calories that you take in. When you go through a period of not eating anything, your body is going to experience changes that can help you access your stored energy better. This can be the changes in your hormones and the activity of your nervous system.

During the fast, you will notice that there are a few changes that occur in your metabolism including:

> • Norepinephrine: The nervous system is going to send this hormone to your stored fat cells. This hormone causes the fat cells to break down into free fatty acids. The body can then take these fatty acids and use them as energy.

> • HGH or human growth hormone: Levels of the hormone can increase like crazy. This hormone can help aid in many processes of the body, including muscle gain and fat loss.

> • Insulin: When you eat any food, your insulin is going to increase. But when you go on a fast, your insulin levels will decrease quite a bit. Lower levels of insulin in the body will help you burn more fat.

Despite what proponents of five to six meals each day say, going on these short-term fasts can actually help you increase the amount of fat that you burn during the day. In fact, two studies found that fasting for a 48-hour time period can help boost your metabolism by up to 14 percent.

The amazing thing about intermittent fasting is that it helps you to affect your hormones in a natural way. As long as your fasting period doesn't last for more than 48 hours, you are not going to cause any negative harm to the body. Instead, you will positively affect your hormones, so they behave in a way that is beneficial to you. You will be better able to regulate your insulin levels, keep your metabolism moving fast, and even help you to feel less hungry throughout the day.

However, you need to be careful with this one. If you go for a period that is too long, such as a 72-hour fast, you can actually suppress your metabolism. Stick with these shorter-term fasts to get the most benefits and the faster metabolism from fasting.

Fasting Is a Great Way to Reduce Your Calories and Lose Weight Naturally

The main reason that intermittent fasts work to help you lose weight is because they make it easier for you to eat fewer calories without feeling deprived. All the protocols for fasting involve skipping meals. Unless you go crazy with compensating for your calories during the eating period, you can take in fewer calories during the day.

According to a review study that was done in 2014, intermittent fasting reduced the body weight of participants by up to 8 percent over a time period that lasted between three to 24 weeks. When looking at this rapid weight loss rate, people were able to lose about 0.55 pounds each week when doing intermittent fasting, but about 1.65 pounds each week when they went on an alternate fasting diet. Those who were in this review also showed that people lost between four to seven percent of their waist circumference, which showed that they also lost belly fat during this time.

These results are impressive and show that alternate day fasting and intermittent fasting can be useful when it comes to losing weight. In addition, the benefits of fasting can go beyond weight loss. It has many benefits on the health of your metabolism and can help expand your lifespan, prevent chronic diseases, and so much more.

While intermittent fasting often doesn't require calorie counting because you can naturally reduce your calories with this method, you may still want to watch your total calories and the types of food that you are eating. Studies have shown that continuous calorie restriction and intermittent fasting have the same results when it comes to weight loss, but intermittent fasting is often seen as much easier to follow.

While some preliminary studies show that intermittent fasting and continuous calorie restriction will give about the same results when it comes to calories burnt and weight loss, many people find that sticking with the intermittent fast is easier. Moreover, when an eating plan is more effective to stick with, people are more likely to follow it and see results.

Intermittent Fasting Can Help You Keep Your Muscle Tone When You Diet

One thing that can happen when you go on a diet is that the body may burn through some of the muscle as well as the fat. However, there are a few studies that show how intermittent fasting can be beneficial to helping you hold onto your muscle, even while you are losing body fat.

With one review study, it was found that doing calorie restriction through intermittent fasting can cause a similar amount of weight loss as continuous calorie restriction. However, one difference is that the former resulted in a smaller reduction in muscle mass through that time.

In the study that looked at calorie restriction, there was about 25 percent of the weight loss that was a result of lost muscle mass. But with intermittent fasting, the amount of weight that was lost to reduced muscle mass was only ten percent. In one of the studies, those who participated would eat the same number of calories as before, but they would just have one large meal in the evening rather than having the calories spread out throughout the day. These participants ended up losing body fat while increasing their muscle mass compared to regular dieting. There were also a ton of other beneficial changes to the health markers in those who did this kind of intermittent fasting.

Intermittent Fasting Not Only Helps with Weight Loss but Also with Making Healthy Eating Easier

One of the best benefits that come with intermittent fasting, in addition to the weight loss and all the health benefits, is that this eating plan is really simple. There are many methods that you can choose to go with; however, all of them are simple and don't contain a lot of hard to follow rules. Simply stick with the eating and fasting windows that are listed in your protocol, and you are going to see some great results.

Compared to some of the other diet plans that you may have tried out in the past, intermittent fasting is going to be simple and easy. You eat at certain times, you avoid eating at others, and you fill your body with lots of healthy nutrients when you can. If you can follow these rules, you will see all the results that you need from intermittent fasting.

Compared to other dieting plans that you can choose, intermittent fasting can provide you with the best results. It naturally works with your body to help you burn fat fast and speeds up your metabolism, so you can burn more calories and lose weight. Add to all this the simplicity of it. It is no wonder that many people choose to go with this eating plan rather than sticking with one of their old dieting plans.

Chapter 3: The Art of Autophagy: How Intermittent Fasting Can Help Clean out the Body

One neat thing that can happen when you are on an intermittent fast is a process that is known as autophagy. This word derives from the Greek word *auto*, which means 'self', and *phagein*, which means 'to eat'. So, if we are looking at the literal meaning of the word, we are looking at a word that means to eat oneself. Of course, this is not exactly what we mean by autophagy.

Instead, we mean that we are looking at the mechanism of the body to get rid of any waste, any old cells, or anything that has broken down once the body doesn't have enough energy to sustain it. It is regulated and orderly and helps the body to stay healthy and not hold onto all the waste that the body releases through your daily life.

Autophagy was first heard about in 1962 when researchers noted that the number of lysosomes in rat liver cells after there was an infusion of glucagon ended up increasing. The lysosomes are the part of the cell that is responsible for destroying stuff. This process was eventually coined as autophagy. The damaged subcellular parts, as well as any unused proteins in the cells, were marked for destruction and then sent over to the lysosomes to help finish up the job.

One of the parts that are important for regulating autophagy is the kinase that goes by the name of mTOR or the mammalian target of rapamycin. When this is activated, it suppresses the process of autophagy. However, when this regulator is dormant, the process of autophagy is promoted and works better.

What Will Activate the Process of Autophagy?

The biggest thing that can activate autophagy is nutrient deprivation. Remember that glucagon is pretty much the opposite of insulin. If the levels of insulin in the body go up, then glucagon is going to go down. The opposite can also be true. If insulin levels go down, then the levels of glucagon will go up. Any time that we eat something, our levels of insulin are going to go up, and it makes it hard for the glucagon because it goes down. If glucagon doesn't have time to elevate at all because you are eating all day long, then you won't be able to have the process of autophagy in the body. Fasting can raise glucagon, which means it is one of the best ways to boost autophagy.

This is the basics of cellular cleansing. The body is going to identify the old and bad cellular equipment in the body and will put a little mark on it for destruction. If all this junk stays in the body and isn't cleaned out, it often affects the aging process in the body.

Not only can fasting help to stimulate this autophagy process, but it can also help in other ways as well. When you fast and stimulate autophagy, you are cleaning out all the old proteins and parts of the cells. In addition, fasting can also stimulate a growth hormone. This hormone will tell the body to start producing the new replacement parts in the body. So, when you go on one of these fasts, you are effectively giving your body a new renovation.

You have to take the time to get rid of all the old stuff before you have a chance to put in any of the new. Think about doing a renovation in your kitchen. If you have an older kitchen that is an eyesore, you must go through it and get rid of all the old cabinets and countertops and everything else to make room for the new stuff. This same idea is important when it comes to the building up of cells in the body. If you just try to build up new cells in the body, without removing all the bad stuff first, it is just going to end up a mess.

Intermittent fasting can really help to handle this. It ensures that you can take care of the body, remove all the old stuff that is there, and then make room for the new. Fasting can provide a natural detox that can improve your health and reverse the aging process, and it is so simple to follow.

A Process That Is Highly Controlled

The process of autophagy is very regulated. If it was able to run out of control, it could be very detrimental to the body, so it is controlled. In the mammalian cells, total depletion of amino acids can be a very strong signal for this process to control, but the role of the individual amino acids can be more variable. On the other hand, the amino acid of the plasma will vary only a little bit. The insulin signals, the growth factor signals, and the amino acid signals are going to converge on the mTOR pathway and will all work to regulate this process.

During autophagy, you can naturally clean out the body. This provides a natural detox that is so good when it comes to your health and weight loss. In a traditional American diet, though, it is very hard to go on a fast. Remember, autophagy can't happen when insulin levels are high. And insulin levels are going to be high if you are constantly eating all the time.

A typical American has a diet that allows them to eat something from the moment they get up until the moment they go to sleep. This makes it hard to let the process of autophagy even start and can cause aging, cancer, Alzheimer's, and other issues.

When you spend time on a fast, you will see that things change. Your levels of insulin will go down, allowing glucagon to increase and the process of autophagy to occur. You have to give your body some time to see this change though. The fast doesn't have to be long, but either a full day fast once or twice a week or a short daily fast can be enough to help you clean out the body, while also creating new cells and giving them room to grow at the same time.

Chapter 4: The Different Types of Fasts That You Can Go On

When we talk about intermittent fasting, there are a few different options that you can consider. Some involve doing a small fast each day while others are full-day fasts during the week. Some of these options are:

The 16/8 Method

This popular method requires a small fast daily that lasts about 16 hours. During that time, you are not allowed to eat any solid food. Options like coffee, water, and other non-caloric beverages can be consumed to help keep you full and ensure that you stay hydrated. After the fast is done, you are given an eight-hour window to eat.

This method is pretty easy to follow. It is as simple as finishing dinner one night and then waiting until lunchtime to eat your next meal. If you get up in the morning, get the kids off to school and do some work, the morning will fly by, and soon it will be time to eat. You can do other variations as well as having an early dinner, so you can eat breakfast, as long as you stay in that eight-hour eating window.

There are also different options that you can choose with this method. Some people need a longer eating window to start out, so they may fast for 14 to 15 hours, and then have their eating window for the remaining hours. No matter how you do it, make sure that your eating window is full of lots of healthy and delicious foods, ones that will keep you full, keep those cravings away, and help you lose weight.

Eat Stop Eat

This method has you pick one to two days during the week where you will do a 24-hour fast. During this time, you are not allowed to eat anything solid. You can enjoy beverages, especially water, non-caloric beverages, and coffee. You have to wait until the fast is over before you can eat anything else. For the other days of the week, you can eat normally, and as healthy as possible.

This method doesn't need to be as complicated as it sounds. You don't have to go from supper one day, miss a meal the next day, and then finally have breakfast two days later. This is technically a 36-hour fast. So instead, you can go from supper one night and then eat the next day at supper. Or you can go from lunch one day to lunch the second, or even breakfast to breakfast. Many people who do the 'eat stop eat' method will go from supper to supper because this helps them to never go to bed hungry.

The 5:2 Diet

This method works like alternate day fasting, but you only go on a fast for two days out of the week. You can pick any two days that you want; just make sure they are not consecutive. During those fasting days, you need to keep your calorie count to 500 or less for the entire day.

There are a few options here. You can choose to take that 500 calories and split it up into two meals. This allows you to still get some food in throughout the day and is sometimes easier for you to accomplish. Others find that when they are fasting, once they start eating, it is hard to stop, and they need to eat more than 250 calories for that meal. These individuals may find that saving the calories and eating all 500 at once is better. They can save the calories for supper, staying in the fast a bit longer, and then splurge a bit more when they finally do get to eat that day.

For the other five days of the week, you can eat normally. Try to stick with a healthy diet with lots of the nutrients the body needs. When you combine a few days a week with only 500 calories and then eat normally during the normal days, you can still end up with a deficit at the end of the week.

The Warrior Diet

The warrior diet follows the same idea as the 16/8 method but takes things a little bit further with a shorter eating window. This diet was originally developed to help weightlifters and bodybuilders burn through any excess body fat and get stronger for competitions, but this doesn't mean that anyone can't give it a try to help lose weight and feel better.

The warrior diet puts the individual on a schedule where they fast for 20 hours during the day. During this time, you can have a few fresh fruits and vegetables, as long as you consume them raw, and you only eat a few hundred calories or less worth of those each day. You should not be getting a ton of calories from this grazing before your eating window. This is only meant to help quell your eating patterns a bit.

For the other four hours of the day, you are allowed to eat. You can choose to split that time up into two meals, or you can have just one big meal to end your day. You need to make sure that you get in all the nutrients that the body needs during this time. Since you are limiting your eating window so much, it is easier to feel full on fewer calories, and your body can spend most of the day in fat burning mode.

The warrior diet is often hard to get started on, especially if you are used to eating all day long and providing your body with a constant supply of glucose. It is a long time to go without eating, and then you have to choose good foods, to provide your body with enough nutrition, which can be difficult. You may want to start with one of the other fasting methods like the 16/8 method to make it easier to start.

The Master Cleanse

The Master Cleanse is usually considered as too restrictive and too long of a fast to fit under the idea of intermittent fasting, but we are going to look at it to see how it is different from intermittent fasting.

The Master Cleanse has gained popularity in the past few years due to many celebrities who have claimed to go on it to lose a lot of weight. The ideas behind this kind of cleanse are often not very healthy, and while you will probably lose a lot of weight, much of it will come back as soon as you start to eat a healthy diet again.

This diet is also called The Lemonade Diet, and it is a liquid only fast. The claim with this fast is that if you stick with it for ten days or so, you will drop weight, clean out your system, and feel more energetic and healthier. It also states that this cleanse can help you curb cravings for unhealthy foods.

During the fast, you can only drink a herbal laxative tea, lemonade, and then a salt water drink for ten days. After the ten days are up, it is fine to add some foods back in slowly, but you will need to take it slowly. Your body has been on low calories for more than a week so bombarding it with a ton of calories is never a good idea. Start the first few days with some soups and a little juice and then move to fresh produce. Slowly move up until you are back to a healthy diet plan.

Since you are taking in fewer calories than before, it's likely that this fast will help you lose weight. However, the ingredients that you can have on this fast are going to be so low in calories that you could lose water weight, muscle tone, and more. And since you are not going to be able to stay on this diet plan forever, it is likely that when you add more calories back into your diet, the weight will come back.

The Master Cleanse is hard and may cause unneeded stress on your digestive system and hormones. It is often better to go with one of the shorter fasts mentioned earlier because they can provide you with all the health benefits that you need without causing harm to your body. If you are worried about getting on a fast and fighting off those cravings, a version of the Master Cleanse can be helpful, but consider doing it for just a few days, rather than ten.

Chapter 5: What Is the Difference Between Intermittent Fasting, Alternate Day Fasting, and Extended Fasting?

As you look at the world of fasting and do some research, you may notice that there are actually many kinds of fasts. Some of these are intermittent fasting methods, but others are unique, and you may wonder how they compare to intermittent fasting. Let's take a look at the difference between intermittent fasting, alternate day fasting, and extended fasting and the benefits and negatives of following each type of fasting.

Intermittent Fasting

This is simple to follow, and there are a few different methods that you can pick from to suit your needs. An intermittent fast requires you to split up your day between eating times and fasting times. The goal is to make your fasting time longer than your eating times. This gives the body time to get into a fasting state, encouraging autophagy and making it easier for you to burn the fat stored in your body.

There are a few different types of intermittent fasting. Some people will spend one or two days a week fasting for a whole day, or do a smaller fast every day of the week, or, like the alternate day fasting (described below), fast three or four days of the week.

All these methods can be effective, and it often depends on the method that works the best for your schedule. These fasts all allow you to take a break from eating all the time, so your insulin levels can stabilize and the natural fat burning and cleaning out process of the body can occur.

The nice thing about intermittent fasting is that it can naturally fit into your current schedule and it doesn't necessarily consist of doing much work. In addition, the fast is short enough that you can get all the health and weight loss benefits without having to worry about entering starvation mode and all the problems that can entail.

Alternate Day Fasting

Alternate day fasting is one of the options that you can choose to help you with intermittent fasting. This method involves fasting every other day of the week. The other days can be regular eating days, and you can enjoy whatever you would like. The most common version of this diet is similar to the 5:2 diet. With this modified version, which can be a bit easier for some people to follow, you are allowed to have 500 calories on your fasting days.

When you see a study done on intermittent fasting, it is most likely to have been done on the alternate day fasting. This type of fasting can be a powerful way to lose some weight while also reducing some of the risks you have for heart disease and can prevent type 2 diabetes.

The basic idea that comes with this type of fast is that you are going to fast on one day, then eat normally on the second. Then you will alternate back and forth between the regular diet days and the fasting days. This means that you only need to place restrictions on what you are eating half the time. During your fasting days, you can drink as much water and other calorie-free beverages as you need to keep yourself hydrated.

If you are following this method, there is an option to modify it if you find it too hard not to eat anything that many days of the week. You can consume up to 500 calories during your fasting days. This still gives you a calorie deficit since it is much less than what you need during the whole week. The benefits that you get with this are going to be similar, regardless of whether you have the calories placed at dinner, lunch, or split up through the day.

While this may seem like an extreme version of intermittent fasting, one that is going to be difficult to do, studies have shown that many people like alternate day fasting and find it easier to stick with compared to regular calorie restriction. Moreover, most of the studies on this kind of fasting focus on the modified version so this can make things even easier.

Extended Fasting

Long-term fasting can often take different forms. The most extreme of these is a dry fast where you don't drink any food or water, but this is often not advisable because not only are you missing out on food, but you are missing out on some of the hydration that you need. There is also a water fast, which means that you can have all the water and hydration that you need, but you won't consume any calories during the fast. Some people may go on a juice fast or even a low-calorie protein fast.

These extended fasts are going to last longer than the other two types of fasts. Alternate day fasting is every other day and can be a form of intermittent fasting. Intermittent fasting is usually 24 hours or less and can either happen a few days a week, every other day of the week, or every day of the week for certain hours. However, with extended fasting, you are going to spend even longer fasting. Often, people will spend a week or more on one of these fasts.

We are going to look at one of the most common extended fasts that you can choose. This one is a water fast and is often done for extreme weight loss quickly or for religious purposes. We will look at the benefits, the negatives, and some of the precautions.

The biggest reason that someone will choose to go on an extended fast is to help with weight loss. If you don't eat anything for an extended period, your body will drop the weight. For the first day of the fast, you are going to see the body use up all the glycogen that is in the liver. Then the body will rely on what it has stored, either fat or protein.

After you get through this first day or so, your body may lose about one to two pounds each day. This comes from using up the protein in the body and shedding some water weight. The body will decide that burning muscle is not a good thing since you need your heart to pump to keep you alive and will work on burning through the stored fat. Since fat is more energy dense for each pound compared to protein, the weight loss may slow down after the first few days. It is still rapid weight loss, though, and can result in one pound every two days.

The problem with this is that once you go back to your old ways of eating, you are most likely to gain all the weight, or at least most of it, back. And there are sometimes dangerous consequences to this kind of fasting. Even a fast that is less than a few weeks can cause issues. This extreme type of fasting can put two stress types on the heart. First, it is going to cannibalize the muscles of the heart to use for fuel. The body is going to try to conserve muscle during a fast, but sometimes it has to sacrifice it to keep you alive, and this can affect the heart.

In addition, strict water fasting can put you at a higher risk for heart failure because when you are on one of these fasts, the intracellular stores of minerals that protect the heart are going to be depleted. This could cause mineral deprivation and can be tragic. In addition, if you get sick during this time, it is harder to fight illness and can put you at risk as well.

Some people who go on very extreme extended fasts may see even more serious effects, and some have even died. This is not very common, and the biggest case of this happening was in 1981 when ten political prisoners went on a fast for 46 to 73 days and starved themselves to death during a hunger strike.

An extended fast can be useful in some cases: it can help you to lose a lot of weight quickly; put the body into ketosis, so it starts to burn off some of the excess fat that is hanging around the body; and, in some cases, helps the individual develop a healthier relationship with food that they can carry forward into the future. However, before you go on one of these fasts, you must make sure you are in good health. Talk it over with your doctor to make sure you are being safe, and make sure that you don't go on an extended fast that is too long.

Chapter 6: Intermittent Fasting and Improved Insulin Sensitivity

Now it is time to move onto some of the benefits that you can get when you decide to implement an intermittent fast. First, we will look at how intermittent fasting can help improve your insulin levels. Insulin is a hormone that the pancreas will produce, and it can play a vital role in helping the body regulate and control your levels of blood sugar. Insulin can be helpful in making sure your blood sugars never go too low or too high.

Despite the bad reputation of insulin, your body does need it to function. The body is going to use sugar, also known as glucose, to function and it gets this from the food you eat. However, the body can't directly absorb this nutrient, and it needs some help. The beta cells that are found in the pancreas will release insulin into your bloodstream to help the sugar get absorbed by the cells and be used as a form of energy. Without this insulin, sugar can't be absorbed properly and will just sit around.

If the body receives more sugar that it needs, insulin will take that sugar and store it in the liver to use later when you need some extra, such as when you are fasting or exercising. Insulin has another job of letting the liver know when it should stop releasing glucose into the blood.

In some cases, the body will not be able to produce enough insulin. Or there could be the problem of insulin having a minimal effect on the cells of the body. When this happens, your levels of blood sugar may get too high. This is a condition that is known as hyperglycemia. This condition can cause many other complications to your health, including loss of consciousness, vomiting, infections, numbness, weight loss, tiredness, hunger, thirst, and frequent trips to the bathroom.

What Does Insulin Resistance Mean?

Insulin resistance is going to occur whenever the cells in your body won't respond to insulin properly and aren't able to absorb the glucose that is in the blood. This is going to force the pancreas to get to work and produce more of the insulin that you need. In some cases, this may get severe enough that you will need to take injections of insulin. This extra insulin is meant to help the cells of the body absorb the glucose that you eat. This issue is a common occurrence in those with type 2 diabetes and prediabetes.

Certain individuals are more likely to suffer from either prediabetes or type 2 diabetes where the body's cells just don't respond to the insulin that is there. When this happens, it can mean that a lot of extra glucose is hanging around in the blood and storing that extra nutrient as body fat. People who might be at a higher risk for these conditions include:

- Those who are on some types of medications, such as HIV medications and antipsychotics.

- Those who suffer from various sleep conditions like sleep apnea.

- Those who are Hispanic, American Indian, Asian American, and African American.

- Those who have had issues with their heart health or who suffered from a stroke in the past.

- Those who have poor levels of cholesterol and high blood pressure.

- Those who don't get enough physical activity into their day.

- Those who already have a family member who suffers from diabetes.

- Those who are 45 years or older.

- Those who are obese or overweight.

There is still research being done on the exact cause of this insulin resistance. However, it is believed that lack of activity and excess weight are the two main factors that can cause this. Helping yourself keep at a healthy weight and making sure that you get up and be active on a regular basis may be the key to preventing this insulin resistance.

How Will an Intermittent Fast Affect My Insulin Levels?

You will quickly find that intermittent fasting can do a great deal of good when it comes to increasing your lipolysis and lowering your levels of insulin. Lipolysis is a process of the fat cells breaking down in the body. When you fast for a longer period, it can reduce the deposits of fat that are in your body. As these deposits get smaller, the cells in the liver and the muscles start to respond more to the insulin that is there.

This can make it so much easier for the insulin and glucose in the body to move into the cells and can decrease your risk of high blood sugar. It can also be good for the cells as well.

When you have lots of food readily available, the body is going to be less sensitive to insulin. The higher insulin levels that are produced to compensate for this will inhibit the secretion of HGH. In fact,

HGH and insulin are going to work in opposing manners. The main role of insulin is to focus on storing energy and pro-inflammatory functions while HGH focuses on optimizing the use of fuel, tissue repair, and stopping inflammation.

When your insulin levels are higher, the HGH levels will be lower. Studies show that elevated insulin levels can help diminish the neuronal autophagy that we talked about earlier. When your body can't go through the process of autophagy, old and damaged cells are going to stick around, and the body will run into trouble functioning the right way.

When the body goes on a fast, it can help to reduce those levels of insulin. The body isn't receiving food, and insulin is only released when there is food that can be turned into glucose and used as energy by the body. Without food, the body won't produce insulin, and the levels go down.

With the traditional way of eating, we often feed the body nonstop, causing our insulin levels to be high. The cells become less sensitive to the insulin because they are bombarded with it all the time. In addition, the higher insulin levels can cause trouble with autophagy occurring and leads to an increase in old and damaged cells in the body.

Fasting can help solve this issue. It turns off insulin production during parts of the day, allowing the cells to have a break. When the cells aren't as bombarded with insulin, it can increase their sensitivity to it later. They will, over time, be better able to absorb the nutrients that you take in due to this change in sensitivity, which is exactly what you want when it comes to preventing or reversing diabetes. You also give the body a chance to lower insulin levels so that autophagy can occur and clean out the body.

If you simply continue to eat nonstop, you are making the problem worse. Insulin will continue to rise, and you will continue to see a reduction in the sensitivity of your cells to insulin. This is how prediabetes and type 2 diabetes end up occurring. Fasting can help give your body a break, to reduce your levels of insulin, so you can see better results with reducing your risk of diabetes.

How Long Do I Need to Do a Fast to Reduce My Levels of Insulin?

Your levels of insulin are going to rise any time you eat. However, the amount that these levels rise will depend on what you eat. The more carbs you take in, the higher your insulin levels and the more likely that sensitivity in the cells will be reduced. These higher insulin levels can easily stay high for a few hours after you eat, and then after you go some time without eating, they will slowly start to fall again.

According to Intensive Dietary Management, your insulin levels will start falling sometime between six to 24 hours after you start fasting as your glycogen starts to get broken down and is used by the body as a source of energy. This phase is going to be known as the post-absorptive phase. After 24 to 48 hours, the body is going to switch over and will enter the gluconeogenesis state.

During this state, the liver is going to take amino acids and start producing new glucose. Then, after 48 to 72 hours of fasting, the body will enter a process of ketosis. This is when your insulin levels will start to really fall low, and the body will turn to fat as its energy source. Through this process, you will see that the easiest way for you to reduce the levels of insulin in your body is to go on a fast and not eat.

Dr. Naiman, who is known for running the Burn Fat Not Sugar website, argues that fasting between 18 to 24 hours is the best because insulin levels are going to see the biggest drop off during this time while you still see the fat breakdown, or lipolysis, increase. However, it appears that going on a fast for a longer period, such as for 24 hours, could have the biggest effect when it comes to reducing your insulin levels.

Therefore, alternate day fasting is so popular. There are many studies out there that show how alternate day fasting can help decrease fat, body weight, and insulin. In one of these studies, published in the US National Library of Medicine, 16 participants, eight women, and eight men, who weren't obese at the start of the study, went on an alternate day fasting schedule for a period of 22 days. During this time, the researchers looked at various numbers to help them see what occurred during the fast, including the resting metabolic rate, body composition, weight, insulin, ghrelin, and fasting serum glucose to name a few items.

The results showed many interesting things. First, most of the subjects lost an average of 2.5 percent of their initial body weight and their insulin levels decreased by 57 percent, plus or minus four percent on average. However, some scores didn't change up, including ghrelin, glucose, and RMR. Hunger didn't seem to decrease on any of the fasting days which showed that some of the participants might run into difficulties if they continued this diet over the long term. To keep this diet going over the long term, it may be best to do the modified version of alternate day fasting to help add in a meal on that fasting day.

Another case study, found in the Journal of Insulin Resistance, followed a patient with type 2 diabetes from Ontario for four months. At the beginning of the study, the patient was fasting for 24 hours three times a week. However, over the course of the study, that patient started to increase their fasting sessions to 42 hours two or three times each week.

When this study was done, the patient had lost 17.8 percent of their body weight, and their waist was 11 percent smaller. However, what was the most surprising effect of this change was that the patient was able to discontinue using insulin treatments at the end of the fast, despite having been on insulin for more than ten years prior.

Although these are small studies, they give a good idea on how effective fasting can be at reducing your levels of insulin and helping you to reduce your risks of developing diabetes in the future. It can even help optimize the levels of insulin in those who already have type 2 diabetes and who are trying to properly manage it for their health. While these results may not be the same for everyone who goes on an intermittent fast, they still provide some insight into how great this eating plan can be.

Chapter 7: Intermittent Fasting and Reduced Levels of Inflammation Throughout the Body

Inflammation is not always a bad thing. It is often the start of the healing process inside the body. While many people strive to reduce inflammation after they suffer an injury, some inflammation, if it is minimal and doesn't stick around for a long time, can be beneficial because it tells the body that it is time to start healing. However, when inflammation is constantly around, or it lasts longer than normal, major health problems can occur.

Inflammation can become a bad thing when it sticks around, and it is going to play a big role in many chronic conditions like cancer, asthma, obesity, and Crohn's disease. Chronic inflammation can be problematic because it can be the start of other issues like back pain, osteoporosis, and arthritis. Add to all this the growing proof that inflammation can cause other issues, such as Alzheimer's, obesity, dementia, and depression. It is no wonder that many people are afraid of inflammation.

There are many different reasons that you may suffer from inflammation, but often it is caused by poor lifestyle choices. It could be from consuming too much processed foods and sugars or not getting enough physical activity in your life. Other issues that could cause this inflammation include gut health problems, exhaustion, and stress.

Is It Possible for Intermittent Fasting to Reduce Inflammation?

There is some evidence that shows how intermittent fasting can be a very effective way to reduce inflammation throughout the body. Research shows how intermittent fasting could have a protective effect against several issues, including inflammation, high insulin levels, and high blood pressure. Intermittent fasting could also help with conditions that increase inflammation, including autoimmune conditions and type 2 diabetes.

In one of these studies, the researcher would feed mice either a high-fat or low-fat diet for a period of ten to 12 weeks. After fasting, the mice who were fed a low-fat diet lost more body weight compared to the other group, did better on learning tasks and memory, and showed more locomotor activity. The mice who were on the low-fat diet also had an improved immune and nervous system function. The conclusion here is that fasting has an anti-inflammatory effect on our bodies, which is something that the high-fat diet may prevent from happening.

Another study looked at those who went on a Ramadan fast. This study was done in 2017 and published in the US National Library of Medicine. It compared 83 people with NAFLD or nonalcoholic fatty liver disease. 42 of these individuals fasted and 41 were the control group who didn't fast. Those who fasted had big reductions in inflammation, insulin resistance, plasma insulin, and glucose compared to the other group.

How Can Intermittent Fasting Help Reduce Inflammation?

There are many ways that intermittent fasting can help reduce inflammation throughout the body. Some of these include:

• Promotes autophagy: We have discussed this briefly, but when the process of autophagy is allowed to occur, the inflammation in the body will go down as it cleans itself out.

• Promotes BHB: Beta-hydroxybutyrate is one of the three main types of ketones that the mitochondria of the liver produce. This one can protect the body against inflammation, improve cognition, can reduce the risk of cancer, and regulates appetite. There are several times when the body is going to produce BHB including:

o When you severely restrict your calories, or you go on a fast.

o You perform high-intensity exercises.

o You consume a supplement that has BHB inside it.

o You consume a salt, such as calcium or magnesium, that can be absorbed easily in the body.

o You follow a ketogenic diet or one that is high fat and low carb.

• Improves your sensitivity to insulin: When the cells are sensitive to the insulin that you produce, they will easily absorb the glucose that is in your food. However, when the sensitivity goes down, or you eat too much of the glucose-producing foods, the cells won't take it up. This glucose sits around the body and can cause a lot of inflammation. Intermittent fasting can help to kick up the sensitivity of the cells to insulin, so they can absorb the glucose and not deal with all the inflammation inside.

• Lowers Leukotriene B4 (LTB4): LTB4 is a proinflammatory lipid that is going to increase inflammation quite a bit. It can play a role in chronic inflammation and can be responsible for many different health conditions, including inflammatory bowel disease, asthma, and rheumatoid arthritis. Research shows that LTB4 can also cause resistance to insulin in mice. Fasting is one way to lower the levels of LTB4 in the body to help reduce some of the inflammation.

• Fights off oxidative stress: This kind of stress occurs when there is a big imbalance between the antioxidants and free radicals in the body. The free radicals are unstable molecules that will oxidize with the other molecules found in your body. This can result in damage to tissues, DNA, and cells and can lead to many inflammatory conditions. These free radicals can be caused by things like:

o Eating too many carbs, sugars, and calories. The body must convert these into energy, and it takes a lot of work. This can lead to more of the free radicals through the body.

o Not getting enough exercise. You need to keep your body in optimal shape to boost your immunity and fight off the oxidative stress.

o Alcohol consumption has been shown to increase inflammation.

o Cigarettes contain many bad chemicals that can increase the risk of oxidative stress.

o Chronic stress has been shown to have a huge negative impact on your overall health, and if it happens often, it can lead to inflammation.

o Various environmental factors. This could include radiation, ozone, and pollution.

What Does the Research Have to Say About All This?

There has been a lot of research done on intermittent fasting, and some of it shows how fasting could help to protect you against inflammation and oxidative stress in the body. One of these studies looked at alternate day fasting and its effects on overweight adults who were suffering from asthma. Ten of the patients were put on a diet where they would fast every other day, or do an alternate day fast, for eight weeks. At the end of this study, those patients showed a huge reduction in the amount of inflammation they had.

In another clinical trial, researchers decided to look at how fasting would be able to change the cells in the body. 24 participants were invited, and they were to practice intermittent fasting for two three-week sessions. During the first of the three-week sessions, the participants went on what was considered a modified intermittent fasting diet. On this, they would alternate between fasting days where they took in 25 percent of their normal caloric intake and feasting days where they would take in 75 percent of their normal calories.

For the second of the three-week sessions, the participants followed that same kind of modified fasting diet, but then they also took some supplements, including an anti-oxidant, vitamin E, and vitamin A.

What the researchers were trying to find out is if fasting would improve oxidative stress and if the stress would produce cells that were stronger in these participants. The researchers also wanted to know if taking any antioxidants would inhibit the cells from getting any stronger because those antioxidants could potentially shelter the cells from oxidative stress and from free radicals in the body.

What the researchers found was that fasting was able to help produce more SIRT3, a gene that is going to help improve cells and can inhibit the production of free radicals. Participants in this study also ended up with lower levels of insulin, which helped protect them against developing diabetes.

One thing that was interesting about this study is that taking vitamin E and C seemed to negate some of the positive benefits the participants had when they went on a fast. The belief here is that these antioxidants sheltered the cells from any oxidative stress. Because of this, the cells couldn't develop any defense mechanisms and become stronger to help them deal with any type of stressful stimuli. If you are using intermittent fasting to help prevent inflammation in the body, it is best just to use that and not add in any supplements or antioxidants – since these seem to protect the cells and makes it hard for them to become any stronger.

As you can see, intermittent fasting can be an effective way to help you reduce inflammation and oxidative stress in the body. It is simple to follow, helps you to reduce many issues that can cause inflammation, and can help you finally get some relief!

Chapter 8: Lowering Triglyceride and Cholesterol Levels

Cholesterol is made up of proteins and fat, or lipids, that produce hormones and help your body to break down fats. Cholesterol has gotten kind of a bad name, but it is something that is needed to help keep the body healthy. However, if you have too much cholesterol, it could cause fatty deposits to build up in your blood vessels. This could increase the risk of cardiovascular problems, including coronary artery disease, stroke, and heart attack.

The levels of your cholesterol will be determined by your diet and your genetics. Most cholesterol is going to be produced in the liver, but then you can also get plenty of it from the foods that you consume. Eating foods that have high levels of trans fat, saturated fats, and cholesterol can make your levels of cholesterol increase. Certain foods naturally have more cholesterol in them, so it is important to watch out for them.

High levels of cholesterol can cause atherosclerosis and health complications. Atherosclerosis is a process that will cause plaque to build up in your blood vessels. This can end up narrowing down the blood vessels and will increase your risks of a stroke and heart attack. In fact, heart disease and heart attacks are one of the leading causes of death in the world. Therefore, it is so important to monitor your cholesterol levels as much as possible.

You also need to watch out for your triglyceride levels. Triglycerides are a type of fat that is found in the body because the body can convert some of the food that you eat into this fat. The body will either use these as energy, or it will store them up in the fat cells to use later. If you store too much of this, it can cause fat to accumulate in the body.

These triglycerides are going to be composed of polyunsaturated, monounsaturated, and saturated fats. Each of these types of fat can create a foundation of monounsaturated fatty acids, polyunsaturated fatty acids, and saturated fats. Since these are a type of fat, they are going to get converted into glycerol and free fatty acids any time that you fast, and then they are used as energy. In comparison, cholesterol, during the fast, will be converted to make certain types of hormones or to repair cells.

Your levels of triglycerides can give you a good indication of what you have eaten recently, but the cholesterol is going to give you an idea of what you have consumed over a long period of time. If you generally eat a healthy diet but went out to celebrate last night, your triglyceride levels will be high, but your cholesterol may be low, for example.

How Fasting Can Affect Your Cholesterol Levels

Research shows how fasting can help reduce your levels of cholesterol and how it may be able to decrease your risks of coronary heart disease. One of these studies looked at whether alternate day fasting was able to reduce the risks of coronary heart disease. In this study, sixteen obese adults, four men, and 12 women participated in a ten-week study. Following eight weeks of treatment, the LDL in the patients was reduced by 25 percent while their triglyceride levels went down by 32 percent. In addition to these numbers, the fat mass, waist size, and body weight of the participants were reduced.

In another 12-week study, researchers looked at how exercise and diet affected HDL and LDL levels in obese adults. Most people who are obese will have a lipid profile that is high in LDL and HDL particles. There were 60 subjects, and they were randomly put into four groups. These four groups included those who did alternate day fasting, those who did calorie restriction, those who exercised and did moderate intensity training three times a week, and those in the control group.

Out of this study, researchers found that both diet and exercise had a similar effect on weight loss in the participants, but this affected HDL and LDL in different ways. Those on the alternate day fast and the calorie restriction group had a five percent reduction in weight loss and an increase in LDL, but there were no changes in HDL. In comparison, those who were in the exercise group lost five percent of body weight and saw improvements in their HDL, but no changes in LDL. What this shows is that it may be best to do a combination of diet and exercise so you can improve both types of cholesterol together.

What Are Some Ways to Lower Your Cholesterol?

- Avoid foods that are high in empty calories: Always pick out foods that are high in healthy nutrients and low in empty calories if you want to lose weight and pick foods that will keep you full so that you can lose weight as well as lower your cholesterol levels.

- Lose weight and add in more exercise: As some of the studies above show, exercise and diet combined can be the best way to help lower your bad cholesterol and increase the good cholesterol.

- Eat more protein and fiber: Protein and fiber can do wonders for keeping you full on fewer calories. Plus, a lot of the sources of these nutrients are low in bad fats that can increase your cholesterol levels.

• Avoid overeating and keep your portions small: Intermittent fasting can help with both. Even if you slightly overeat after your fast, the amount is not going to overcompensate for the calories that you missed. And since your eating window is usually smaller, it will be easier for you to keep your portions under control.

• Grilling, boiling, or baking your meals: Deep fat frying and other options than the three listed above can add lots of extra bad fats to your diet, which will increase your cholesterol levels. Try to use healthy cooking methods.

• Do an intermittent fast: Many people who go on an intermittent fast find that it is easier to control their calories and lose weight, which can be important to lower your cholesterol levels. It works the same in many studies as calorie restriction, but for most people, the intermittent fast is easier to maintain.

Chapter 9: Intermittent Fasting and Your Heart Health

So far, we have spent some time talking about the amazing benefits that can come with intermittent fasting. We have even talked about some of the ways that fasting can help improve the health of your heart, such as by lowering your cholesterol levels and reducing inflammation. Just by increasing your insulin sensitivity, intermittent fasting can help reduce your risk of heart disease by 93 percent.

When it comes to looking just at the heart and how healthy it is, many experts look at a variety of factors, including inflammatory markers, blood pressure, triglycerides, and cholesterol levels. And it just happens that intermittent fasting can help reduce all these risk factors. Let's look at how intermittent fasting can really help improve your heart health so that you can live a long and happy life.

How Does Intermittent Fasting Help with Circulation and Healthy Hearts?

Intermittent fasting can be very effective at reducing your risk of circulatory and heart disease. Cardiovascular diseases are one of the leading causes of death in the world, with one in six deaths in the United States attributed to heart disease and one in 19 deaths due to a stroke. Many people wrongly assume that heart disease only occurs in men, but women can be just as much, if not more, at risk of this disease.

There are a variety of risk factors that can lead to cardiovascular disease. Some of these include:

- Being overweight. This is particularly concerning if your waistline is larger and you carry more weight around your middle.

- Lack of exercise.

- Poor diet.

- Diabetes.

- Insulin resistance and a high level of glucose in the blood.

- High blood pressure.

- Smoking has been shown to cause several issues with your heart health. The chemicals that are found in cigarettes can easily cause the blood vessels to narrow, forcing the heart to pump blood harder than before.

Fasting can help with some of these risk factors. For example, it can help you to lose weight so that your weight and your waistline are no longer a big issue. It can help lower your blood pressure, reduce the risk that you have for diabetes, and can reduce insulin resistance. Fasting can even help you get on a healthier diet because your cravings for processed and junk foods will be reduced. If you add in a healthy lifestyle to this as well, you may be able to stop smoking and add in more exercise to help with those risk factors as well.

A Look at How Cardiovascular Disease Can Develop

Cardiovascular disease is a pretty general term that is used to discuss all of the diseases that can occur to your circulation and your heart. It can include coronary heart disease, like a heart attack or angina, heart failure, and even stroke. These diseases are all going to be caused when fatty deposits are allowed to build up in the arteries, a process that is known as atherosclerosis.

The exact cause of this is not always certain. Many people originally thought that it was obvious that having higher levels of fat in the blood would be the culprit of this issue. However, scientific research has shown that this is too easy, and it may not always be the case. The exact kinds of fats that you consume will be the important part. In addition, the amount of inflammation that is found in the arteries may be a factor as well. Carrying an excess amount of fat around the internal organs and having issues with resistance to insulin can also increase your risk of developing this condition.

What is known is that once fats build up in the arteries, they become narrower and stiffer. The result of this is an increase in your blood pressure because it takes more pressure to get the blood through your narrowed arteries. If this narrowing occurs too much, then there can be problems like angina, pain when walking, and even heart attacks. The heart is working hard to pump blood throughout the body, but if the arteries get completely blocked, then the organs, including the heart, won't be able to get the blood that they need to function.

This kind of health concern is going to occur over time, with an unhealthy lifestyle and diet. Many people may not realize the extent of their issues and will wait until it is too late to do something that will make it better. It is much better to work on a healthier lifestyle and diet as early as possible to ensure that you don't have to deal with any of the many cardiovascular diseases that can harm your body.

Is Intermittent Fasting Able to Reduce My Risk of Developing Cardiovascular Disease?

The good news is that many studies have found that intermittent fasting can improve the risk factors for cardiovascular disease. This means that when you are on a fast, you can reduce your risks of developing one of these diseases. Some risk factors, such as insulin resistance, cholesterol, blood pressure, and weight (particularly fat that is around your waist), can all be improved with intermittent fasting.

Individuals who went on a 24-hour fast just once a month were less likely to be diagnosed with coronary artery disease. This is based on a study of 448 people in Utah and those who fasted that was also suffering from type 2 diabetes. Imagine the changes that could happen if these individuals chose to fast for more than one day a month, such as doing the 5:2 diet or an alternate day fasting schedule. Their risk of developing cardiovascular disease may be even lower.

In addition, there were studies done on obese and overweight women who were asked to fast every other day for eight weeks. These participants were allowed to have about 500 calories a day on their fasting day. After the eight weeks were over, these women had lost weight and reduced their waist size, decreased their LDL and cholesterol, lowered their blood pressure, and more.

In a further study, it was found that these same kinds of improvements to cardiovascular health were also seen in people whether they ate on the traditional diet most Americans follow or a low-fat diet on their non-fasting days. Moreover, other studies that look at alternate day fasting have confirmed these benefits to the health of your heart.

Another research study showed that overweight women who did a semi-fast for two days a week, which meant they could eat up to 600 calories on their fasting days, had a reduction in insulin resistance, blood pressure, triglycerides, total and LDL cholesterol, inflammation, and leptin. This shows that whether the women went on an alternate day fast or the 5:2 diet, they saw results that could improve the health of their heart.

Studies have also been done on daily fasting during Ramadan. These studies show that there was an improvement in cardiovascular risks with this type of fasting as well. Often, this form of fasting is not going to be used for the health benefits, though, and is done to follow a religion. Some studies may not encourage this form of fasting to keep you healthy for the long term.

To get some of the good benefits that come from intermittent fasting, you must take the time to eat a diet that is healthy and wholesome. If you go on one of these fasting choices and then spend your time eating a lot of junk and processed foods, it isn't going to help your risk of developing cardiovascular disease, and you will be in just as much trouble as before.

The exact way that intermittent fasting can cause beneficial changes to your cardiovascular risk is still unknown. However, it seems like some of the key factors include helping the individual to lose weight, improve their insulin resistance, and inflammation. The reduction in waist size can be a good indicator that you are heading in the right direction when it comes to reducing your risk of cardiovascular disease. If you have a large risk for cardiovascular disease or you have some of the risk factors discussed above, then it may be time to consider going on a 5:2 diet or an alternate day fast to help you get some results to cut down on your cardiovascular risk.

Chapter 10: Intermittent Fasting and Cancer

One benefit that you can get from intermittent fasting that may be surprising is that it can help protect you from, and fight against, cancer. Studies indicate that fasting can help reduce some of the side effects that come from chemotherapy, improve immunity, slow down the growth of cancerous tumors, and increase survival rates. This benefit still needs more research, but so far, it looks like intermittent fasting can be beneficial and safe for most cancer patients if it is done under the supervision of your doctor or medical professional.

How Can Intermittent Fasting Help Me Fight Cancer?

Fasting can help you fight cancer because it activates the immune system of the body. The immune system is designed to help find and then eliminate anything foreign that is present and could harm your health. However, it is not as effective at finding and then eliminating abnormal cells in the body, such as cancer cells. Intermittent fasting may be just what your immunity needs to become more effective at getting rid of these abnormal cells.

Research that was conducted at the University of Southern California showed that mice who fasted when they received chemotherapy ended up responding more favorably to treatment compared to mice who just went through chemo on its own. The mice that were on a fast produced more of the immune system cells, specifically the T cells and B cells, that were able to target and destroy both tumor cells and breast cancer cells. In addition, fasting can be helpful in making the drugs for chemotherapy more effective and could slow down the spread of cancer to other areas.

Researchers also found that going through many rounds of fasting, or at least more than one, could be enough to slow down the growth of human neuroblastoma, glioma, melanoma, and breast cancer. In some cases, it appears that fasting may be as effective as chemotherapy in treating some types of cancer in some patients.

One study on this had mice who were dealing with human ovarian cancer. The ones who had this and went on a fast ended up living longer than those who didn't fast. In fact, up to 20 percent of the mice who had a deadly form of children's neuroendocrine cancer was cured after doing several rounds of fasting combined with chemotherapy. Another 40 percent of mice showed the lesser spread of same cancer when they combined the two treatments together. In that same study, all the mice who only underwent chemotherapy died.

While studies are limited on how intermittent fasting can affect humans, one study has taken the time to look at the effectiveness, as well as the safety, of fasting while on chemotherapy. For this study, 20 patients with cancer were divided into three groups. One group fasted for 24 hours, one for 48, and the last for 72 hours before chemotherapy. The results of this showed that fasting helped to reduce insulin-like growth factor 1, which is a growth factor that has been linked to certain cancers. Even when the patients went back to their regular diet, the effect from the fast continued for 24 hours after the chemotherapy session ended.

Another neat thing to consider is that individuals who have Laron syndrome, which is a disorder that inhibits IGF-1 also have lower risks of developing diabetes and cancer compared to the general population. This is a similar thing that can happen when patients undergo a fast before chemotherapy. This fasting also helped limit DNA damage and less toxicity in healthy tissues after the chemotherapy treatment was done. The longer fasts seemed to be more effective.

In addition to all the great benefits and the effectiveness of fasting along with chemotherapy, patients who went on the fast found that they didn't undergo severe side effects. At worst, they suffered from dizziness, headaches, and fatigue, which could also happen from the chemotherapy treatment. They had no signs of malnutrition.

Can Fasting Help with Breast Cancer?

Breast cancer patients may be able to benefit from fasting as well. There is evidence that doing a fast or dealing with calorie restriction can help starve out the cancer cells and makes them respond better to chemotherapy. In addition, fasting could boost the immunity of the individual so it can fight off tumor growth and prevent cancer from spreading through the body.

In one study, researchers put mice who had breast cancer on a diet that mimicked a fast, one that was low in sugar, protein, and calories. The mice on this fast had their calories cut in half on the first day, and then the next three days their calories were cut by 9.7 percent. After four days of this diet, the mice were allowed to eat in a normal way for ten days before going on the fast again. This repeated a few times.

Mice who went on this fasting diet had reductions in the cell growth of their breast cancer, even though they didn't go on chemotherapy in that time. Their cancer cells became more sensitive to chemotherapy drugs as well, and their bodies were more effective at finding, targeting, and then destroying tumor growth. After three rounds of this fasting cycle, along with the doxorubicin chemotherapy drugs, the white blood cells of the mice increased by 33 percent. This is an important thing to note since these white blood cells are needed to help the body fight cancer.

But what about the results in humans? One study that was done through the University of California looked at whether daily fasts could help reduce the risks and recurrence of breast cancer. The study took self-reported data from 2,413 women who had early-stage breast cancer between 1995 and 2007. The participants ranged in ages between 27 to 70, and they would fast for an average of 12.5 hours a night.

The women in this study who fasted for 13 hours or less each night ended up having a higher risk of breast cancer recurrence compared to the women who fasted over 13 hours each night. For every increase of two hours in the duration of a nightly fast, there was lower blood sugar levels and a longer duration of nighttime sleep. The report also noted how fasting could help protect against heart disease and type 2 diabetes.

Can Fasting Help Reduce the Side Effects of Chemotherapy?

In addition to helping you fight cancer, fasting can help you get through the side effects of chemotherapy easier. In one study that was done, cancer patients who fasted for a maximum of five days and then had a normal diet before treatment reported that they had fewer side effects compared to those who didn't fast before treatment. They also reported less gastrointestinal issues, less weakness and fatigue, reduced cramps and numbness, fewer headaches, and no vomiting. Moreover, the fasting didn't make them lose an unsafe amount of weight or interfere at all with their treatment.

However, there are a few concerns that have come with intermittent fasting for a cancer patient. The biggest one is that it may cause additional weight loss in a patient who is already at risk for weight loss. While weight loss is good for someone who is obese or overweight, in a cancer patient, it is not a good thing.

Some patients may also have issues with dizziness, headache, weakness, and fatigue because of fasting. And since the patient is already dealing with being in a weaker state due to their treatments, this may make things worse. Therefore, patients who are considering using a fast during their cancer treatment should discuss this option with a doctor before they start. If the doctor and the patient think this is a good option, then the patient must make sure that they start with a shorter fast and slowly extend the duration to see whether the effectiveness is increased.

If a cancer patient is going to go on a longer fast, one that is more than a day or two, then this fast needs to be monitored by a doctor. This will ensure that the patient is getting the nutrition that they need during the fast and that this fast won't mess with their treatment at all. When the patient is not on a fast, they should make sure they eat a well-balanced diet that has a ton of nutrition and whole foods, as well as lower the consumption of refined carbs and eat more protein.

More research needs to be done to help determine whether fasting can be an effective way to help treat cancer and to make sure that the side effects of chemotherapy and other cancer treatments are kept to a minimum. However, with the animal studies and a few reviews that have been done so far, fasting may be the answer that many cancer patients have been waiting for.

Chapter 11: Intermittent Fasting and Epilepsy

Fasting has been used for centuries to help naturally treat the body for many conditions. And now, it may be possible to use intermittent fasting, especially when it is combined with the ketogenic diet, as an effective way to help fight epilepsy. While studies are still out on whether intermittent fasting can help epilepsy effectively on its own, it is very effective when it works with the ketogenic diet.

Early evidence has shown that abstaining from carbs and going on a water fast could help reduce the frequency of epileptic seizures for more than half the patients who were given the fasting based therapy, according to research that has been done at Johns Hopkins University. This is a powerful look at the fact that intermittent fasting may be able to help treat epilepsy, especially for children who rely on medication to provide them some relief from epilepsy.

What Is Epilepsy?

Epilepsy is a chronic disorder where unprovoked and recurrent seizures are normal. A person who suffers epilepsy is classified as one who has two unprovoked seizures that weren't caused by some reversible or known medical condition. For example, if someone had a seizure because their blood sugars got low or they were having withdrawals from alcohol, then they would not be considered epileptic.

The seizures that occur in epilepsy can be related to family tendency and brain injury in some cases, but often the cause is not known. Many people who suffer from this disorder may have more than one type of seizure and other neurological problems.

Although the symptoms of these seizures can affect any part of the body, the events that cause the seizures, including the electrical events, are going to occur in the brain. The location of that event, how far it spreads, and how much of your brain is going to be affected can all have effects on the individual. Sometimes the seizure is smaller and won't cause many issues, but over time, these instances often get worse, and the side effects will grow.

The Ketogenic Diet and Fat Burning

The ketogenic diet is very different from the traditional diet plan that most Americans follow. While many Americans follow a diet that is all about eating lots of carbs and plenty of processed foods, the ketogenic diet relies more on eating lots of healthy fats and keeping the carb content down as much as possible.

As the body switches off from eating carbs and having a constant source of easy glucose to use as fuel, it instead starts to rely on fat as its main source of energy. The body will then start to enter ketosis. The ketones that are produced from that is going to trigger some small biochemical changes in the brain, changes that can be very beneficial to patients who have epilepsy. Trials, as well as observations, show how the ketogenic diet can help at least half of the epilepsy patients who decide to try it and 20 percent of patients are going to see some huge improvements.

While more studies need to be done to see if the ketogenic diet can make changes in the brain that can benefit those with epilepsy, early research shows that the process that goes on during the ketogenic diet can actually help those with this disorder. It is a simple change to make and can definitely help one to avoid seizures.

Fasting May Be a Good Stand-Alone Therapy for Epilepsy

In another study that was done at Johns Hopkins University, there was further evidence of the benefits of using the ketogenic diet along with periodic fasting. This study also showed that these two approaches can complement each other and that using them together can provide the best results. A pediatric neurologist from Johns Hopkins University, Adam Hartman, explains that the current evidence suggests that fasting is not just enhancing the effects of the ketogenic diet in epileptic patients, but it could also be enough to change up the metabolism of children with epilepsy and could be used as a stand-alone therapy for some patients.

In the current study, researchers tested children who went on just the ketogenic diet on its own, and they achieved only moderate results. The children then went on a fast along with the ketogenic diet, and at the end of this, four out of six children who were tested reported that they had fewer seizures.

This helps to prove that fasting may be a good stand-alone treatment for children who are suffering from epilepsy and drug-resistant. The latest study shows that even those who only saw a little bit of relief with the ketogenic diet were able to see some significant results when they started to introduce periodic fasting to the mix as well. Hartman and other researchers plan to focus studies in the future on determining how intermittent fasting can affect seizures and whether fasting would be an effective method to help control certain types of seizures.

Chapter 12: Intermittent Fasting and Improving Your Mind and Preventing Neurodegenerative Diseases

Anything that you do that is good for your body is bound to be good for the brain as well. Intermittent fasting has been shown to improve a variety of metabolic features that are super important when it comes to the health of your brain. This can include things like reducing inflammation, reducing issues with insulin resistance, reducing blood sugar levels, and reducing oxidative stress throughout the body.

There have been several animal studies that show how intermittent fasting can help increase how fast nerve cells can grow. The faster that these nerve cells can grow, the easier it is for the brain to stay sharp and focused no matter what you are working on. Moreover, intermittent fasting can increase the levels of BDNF, or brain-derived neurotrophic factor, in order to fight off various brain problems such as depression. It is no wonder that intermittent fasting is recommended for improving the brain.

There are so many great benefits that come from following an intermittent fast. Many people will see a reduction in some neurodegenerative diseases, an increase in their focus and concentration, and so much more. Let's take a closer look at how intermittent fasting can help protect your brain!

How Intermittent Fasting Helps to Improve the Way That Our Brains Function

One of the most common things that people want to improve on is their concentration and focus at work and in other parts of their life. Fatigue, brain fog, and an inability to keep themselves on task can be common symptoms that people in all industries face each day. Add in some issues like weight gain, high insulin levels, and high blood sugars and our ability to concentrate on the task at hand diminishes further.

Intermittent fasting may be the answer that you are looking for if you need to fight off brain fog and fatigue and you want to be able to concentrate and focus. One recent study showed that when overweight mice went on an intermittent fast, it helped them much better with learning and memory scores. There was also a big improvement in the structural function of their brains. It is a nice combination; a slimmer waistline and better brain function all rolled into one package!

What this means is that by going on an intermittent fast, even by fasting a few days a week, you are greatly improving the overall functioning of your brain. You are clearing out the brain so that it can remember more so that it can focus, and so that concentration is easier than ever before.

Intermittent Fasting and Alzheimer's Disease

Alzheimer's disease is one of the most common neurodegenerative diseases in the whole world. There is no cure available for this disease right now, so the best thing to do is learn how to prevent it in the first place. In one study that was done on rats, it was shown that intermittent fasting might be able to delay Alzheimer's in those who don't have it and reduce the severity in those who already suffer from the disease.

In a series of reports that were done, a lifestyle intervention that had short-term fasts done every day was able to help improve the symptoms of Alzheimer's in nine out of ten patients. In addition, several animal studies suggest that fasting may be able to help with some other neurodegenerative disease, such as Huntington's and Parkinson's disease.

Helps Fight off Depression

Depression and other low mood disorders are quickly rising throughout the world. In fact, this has become such a big issue that the World Health Organization predicts that by 2030, depression is going to be the leading cause of disease burden throughout the whole world. More people than ever are fighting off depression and other mood disorders, and this could be a major problem.

One root cause of depression and low mood could be chronically high insulin and blood sugar levels. The hormones that are affected by these two things, which can also lead to a rise in type 2 diabetes, are also going to affect the hormones that are in control of our moods. With the average sugar consumption at 160 pounds per year per person, it is no wonder that this is a big issue that many people are facing right now.

The best thing to do is work on reducing your high blood sugar and insulin levels. We have already shown how intermittent fasting can help make this happen. By going on a fast and changing up some of the hormones in the body during the process, while also reducing the amount of sugar and refined carbs we take in, not only are we reducing our risk of type 2 diabetes, but we are also working on helping to improve our mood and fight off depression.

Fasting May Be Able to Protect the Brain Against Disease

In addition to all the benefits that we have discussed in this guidebook, fasting may have the power to help protect your brain against various degenerative illnesses. Researchers from the National Institute of Ageing have found evidence that states how periodic fasting or fasting for just one or two days each week, may protect your brain from the effects of Parkinson's, Alzheimer's and other ailments.

When you reduce the number of calories that you take in, it may help your brain. However, doing regular calorie restriction may not be enough to make this happen. It is much better to go on an intermittent fast, or periodically cut out meals in your week, rather than just restricting your calories. Then implement some days where you can eat as much as you want. What this means is that timing is a very crucial element when it comes to how well you can protect your brain.

Cutting daily food intake to about 500 calories for that day, which is going to be a small meal, for two days out of the week, can have some beneficial effects on your brain and how strong it can stay. It is as simple as adding one or two fasting days to your week, and then eating as normally as possible the rest of the week so that you can protect against some neurodegenerative diseases in the body.

Many scientists have known for a long time that eating a diet that is lower in calories can help you lead a longer life. Mice and rats that were raised on restricted amounts of food were able to increase their lifespan 40 percent or more compared to those who didn't restrict their calories. And this same effect has been seen in humans.

But now research is taking this idea a little bit further. It is now argued that by having an occasional fast and not eating as much for one or two days during the week is not going to cause early death or even ill health. However, it could help delay the onset of conditions that could affect the brain, even for conditions like stroke, Parkinson's and Alzheimer's.

The reason that this may work is that the growth of neurons in the brain may be most affected when you reduce the amount of energy that you take in. The amounts of the messaging chemicals between two cells will be boosted when you sharply reduce the number of calories that you consume. These chemical messengers are going to play an important role in boosting the growth of neurons in the brain, something that would be able to counteract how impactful Parkinson's and Alzheimer's are.

The link between boosting cell growth in the brain and reductions in the amount of energy you take in may seem unlikely, but there are some evolutionary reasons for believing in this. In the past, when resources were scarce, our ancestors would need to scrounge around and find food. Those who had brains that could respond well to this, the ones who could remember where promising sources of food were or how to avoid predators, would be the ones who got to the food and survived. This is how this link was developed.

Currently, more studies need to be done on the effect, and researchers, including those at Johns Hopkins University, are getting ready to take it further. They are preparing to study how fasting can impact the brain through MRI scans and other techniques. If the results come back the way that most studies have shown so far, it is possible that the missing link to protecting your brain and your mental health is intermittent fasting.

Chapter 13: Are There Any Negative Side Effects of Going on an Intermittent Fast?

Below are some of the negative side effects of going on an intermittent fast:

- Feeling full after you break your fast and eat.

Our bodies generally follow an unhealthy eating plan. We are used to eating at least three big meals a day and then lots of snacks any time that we feel a bit hungry, when we get near a mealtime, or just have a craving. Because we are used to eating that often, the body learns to expect food at certain times. The ghrelin hormone is responsible for making us feel hungry, and it is set up to peak during the main meal times. It is often regulated by the food that we take in.

- Becoming really obsessed with your eating and fasting windows.

When we decide to go on a fast, the ghrelin levels are still going to peak at the same times that they did before. Even though we aren't eating, and we are going to be just fine moving our meal times around, these levels will peak at breakfast, lunch, and dinner, and we will feel very hungry when they do. Often, days three to five of the fast are going to be the hardest. If you can stick with this for a week or so and adjust your body and the ghrelin levels to eating at different times, the hunger will naturally go away.

- Lots of cravings and hunger.

One option that you can try out when you want to fight off those hunger pains and make sure that you don't give in during your fasting window is to make sure that you take in a lot of water during that time. Water can help fill up the stomach and make you feel more alert. And for some people, the action of just putting something in their mouth to eat, or in this case drink, when they are hungry, can be enough to make the hunger pains go away.

If you need something that is a bit different than water to enjoy during your fasting time to get rid of hunger, you can consider black coffee or drinking some tea. This can help to curb your hunger. Keep yourself busy as well to help you not think about the hunger as much. You can work out, clean the house, or just find something that you enjoy doing.

When it is time to get back to your eating window, you need to make some plans. You must make sure that this time is full of healthy nutrients, and that you are taking in enough calories so that you can fill up. This will easily make a difference in how much hunger you feel during your fasting period.

- Heartburn

- Headaches

As your body gets used to going on an intermittent fast, there are times when the body will experience a dull headache, one that isn't constant but comes and goes. There are different reasons that this may happen, including dehydration if you don't make sure you are drinking enough fluids during your fasting window. It is a good idea to monitor your fluids and always keep a water bottle nearby. When you aren't eating, it is easy to forget that you need to drink, and dehydration and the headaches that accompany it can sneak up on you.

Not only can dehydration cause headaches, but you could experience headaches because of a decrease in your blood sugar levels. Some people experience more stress hormones released in the brain when they decide to fast as well. The good news is that these go away quickly. Just make sure that you drink plenty of water during the day, keep some painkillers around, and take it slowly for the first few days.

- Brain fog in the beginning.

- Can negatively affect the hormones of women.

Some women find that they are going to react negatively to the changes in the amount they eat. For some women, this is not a big issue, and they can change the way that they eat without many issues to start with. However, for some women, changing up the way they eat and any sign that they are going into starvation mode can cause issues with their hormones and can slow down the metabolism.

We will talk about this topic more in a future chapter. Women are often very sensitive to changes in the way that they eat. To preserve the reproductive system, women are going to respond differently to these fasts compared to men, and they need to be careful about how they go on one of these fasts to start with.

- Fatigue

During the first few days, and up to a week, that you are on an intermittent fast, you may feel overly tired. Many people worry that they are doing the fast the wrong way or that it isn't for them because they are so tired when they first get started. The important thing here is just to keep going with the fast and realize that feeling tired in the beginning is completely normal.

When you think about everything that happens when you are on a fast, it shouldn't surprise you as much that you feel so tired at first. With your traditional diet, your body relies much on processed carbs and sugars that are turned into glucose in the body. Glucose is a very easy source of energy, one that the body will actively search for. However, our bodies don't effectively burn through the glucose that we eat, and much of it gets stored as body fat, even as we crave more of it.

With intermittent fasting, we take away that easy source of energy for longer periods of time. The body must learn how to find good sources of energy that aren't glucose to keep us up and running, and this can be hard. For some who had poor eating habits before the fast, it can be hard for the body to know what to go after for fuel.

While the body searches around for the energy that it needs, it is going to be tired. You are going to feel worn down and like you just want to sleep all day long. But it will only take the body a few days before it will start to use the stored glycogen or the stored body fat as fuel, and you will get the energy back. Until that time, take it easy, avoid being around anything that will stress you out or cause you to be irritable (high irritability and low tolerance for stress are common while fasting), and you will be just fine.

For the most part, these negative side effects are just going to be temporary. As the body adjusts to this new form of eating, you will get used to them and won't have to deal with them as much. Just stick it out, and after a week or so on a fasting regimen, you are going to notice a big difference with most side effects gone.

Chapter 14: Men vs. Women – Why Women Should Fast Differently Than Men

Following an intermittent fast can be a great way to help you increase your metabolism, reduce your calories, and lose weight while improving your health all at once. There are many ways that you can go on an intermittent fast, and with all those methods, it's easy for everyone to get on this fast and make it work for their lifestyle. However, women often have to follow some special rules when they go on an intermittent fast to avoid sensitivities to these eating changes that can mess with their hormones and cause problems.

The way that men and women fast will be different, and many times, women will need to take caution and be careful when they decide to fast.

Many women have been worried about going on an intermittent fast because they are worried about issues with metabolic disruptions, menstrual periods, and more from this kind of fasting. Thus, women are going to respond differently to men with these fasts.

This doesn't mean that women aren't able to see results though. It just means that you need to be careful about the way that you fast, and take it slowly, to get the best results. This chapter is going to look at some of the basics that you can follow as a woman on an intermittent fast to get the best results.

As a woman, when you decide to go on an intermittent fast, you must be careful about the method you choose, how much you fast, and the number of calories and nutrition that you take in each day. Women are often sensitive to changes in their diet and even when they get enough nutrition and calories while fasting, the longer periods of not eating may adversely affect them.

Women can still go on an intermittent fast and see some great results, but they do need to take some extra precautions to make sure they are doing it in a manner that is safe and effective for them. For some women, these precautions aren't necessary, and they will be able to go on a fast and not have any negative effects. For other women, this chapter will help them to make sure that they listen to their bodies and stay safe while they are on their fast.

What Happens to the Hormones of Women During Fasting?

Intermittent fasting may not seem like a big deal to most people. They may think that getting into it and experimenting a bit isn't going to make that big of a difference. But for some women, these small decisions can have a huge impact. The hormones in women that are responsible for regulating key functions in women, including ovulation and reproduction, can be sensitive regarding the energy that you take in.

In both genders, the hypothalamic-pituitary-gonadal axis, which is the cooperative functioning of three endocrine glands, can act like an air traffic controller. First, your hypothalamus is going to release a hormone that is known as GnRH. This is then going to tell your pituitary gland to release the LH hormone and the FHS hormone.

These two hormones are going to act on the gonads of the individual, which would be either the ovaries or the testes. In women, this means that these hormones are going to trigger the production of progesterone and estrogen, both of which are needed to help release a mature egg and to help support a pregnancy. For men, these hormones are going to trigger the production of testosterone and sperm production.

This reaction is supposed to happen at a specific time to help the cycle in women stay as regular as possible. To make this happen, the pulses of GnRH must be timed so that everything goes at the right time. However, the problem comes in because these pulses are very sensitive to factors in the environment. And if you don't pay attention to your body and what is going on, these things can sometimes be thrown off through fasting. Even a short-term fast can end up causing many issues for women.

Why Does Fasting Seem to Affect Women More Than Men?

Many studies are unsure about why intermittent fasting affects women more than men. One thought is that it has to do with the levels of kisspeptin in women versus men. This is a molecule neurons use to communicate with each other. This hormone is going to stimulate the production of GnRH in both sexes, and it will have a very high sensitivity to insulin, leptin, and ghrelin hormones that are responsible for regulating hunger and satiety.

One interesting thing is that females produce higher levels of this hormone compared to men. And the more of this hormone in the body, the higher the sensitivity to any changes in energy balance. This may be a good clue as to why many women have trouble going into one of these fasts.

For many women who go on a fast, the best solution that you can try out is to limit the amount of time that you go on a fast to start with.

70

Doing options like either the 5:2 diet or the 16/8 diet are often best, but women should avoid options like the warrior diet.

Are There Any Times When I Should Stop Doing an Intermittent Fast?

Remember that many women are going to be sensitive to changes in eating. While most women can avoid issues simply by slowly entering their intermittent fast, other women may find that intermittent fasting is not for them and they need to try something else. When certain symptoms begin, it is the body's way of telling you that things need to change. Many of these symptoms can lead to serious conditions and health concerns in the future. Some of the signs that intermittent fasting is causing worse than good and that it is time to stop your fasting include:

- You are always cold and can't warm yourself up.

- You notice that your digestive system has slowed down.

- You have no interest in a romantic life, especially if you had a good romance life before the fast.

- Your heart is going to feel like it is making strange beats. Watch out for any rapid beats at random times.

- You have lots of mood swings, and they seem like they are all over the place.

- You notice that when any stress comes up in your life, your tolerance is low, and you just can't seem to handle it at all.

- If you end up getting injured during your time trying out a fast, and you have a lot of trouble healing. In addition, you catch a bug and have trouble fighting it off, no matter what is going around.

- When you finish up with a workout while fasting and are struggling to recover from it. If you used to work out and you start to have trouble with recovering once you start fasting, that is something to watch out for as well.

•You notice that your skin is very dry when you fast and nothing seems to help.

•You see that your hair is falling out.

•It is hard for you to fall asleep and even when you do fall asleep, it is hard for you to stay asleep at night.

•You notice that your menstrual cycle is changing. It may be irregular for more than one month, or you notice that you miss your cycle for a few months in a row (and you are not pregnant).

If you start to notice that a few of these conditions are affecting you, then it may be time to make some changes to your fasting schedule. If you are on an alternate day fast, then maybe move back to the eat stop eat method or 16/8 method to help you lose weight. These are easier on the system and won't affect your hormone levels at all. If you were already on one of those, then it may be time to stop intermittent fasting altogether.

Chapter 15: What Should I Expect When I Get Started with Fasting?

Once you have gotten started with fasting, you may be nervous about what to expect. Most of us have rarely ever missed a meal unless we were sick, and we have spent most of our lives being told that fasting is very bad for our health. Even with knowing all the great health benefits that have been discussed in this guidebook, it can still be a little hard to understand what is going to happen when you start your fast.

For the first few fasts that you undertake, the situation may be difficult. If you can get through the first two or three, then things get easier, but be ready for a rough couple of days as you start to adjust. The hunger that bothers you, in the beginning, will start to dissipate a bit and can be quelled with the help of a drink of water. You may also deal with a few other issues, such as headaches and heartburn like we talked about before, but these often disappear after a few fasts.

Some people are going to experience more issues with their fast compared to others. No one is quite sure why some people have bigger problems, but it may have to do with the diet that you had before you began fasting. One cause of fasting being more difficult for some compared to others is a phenomenon that is known as metabolic inflexibility. This is when the body has become so used to that constant supply of carbs and sugar from food that it is out of practice, turning to our fat stores for energy, and the side effects can hit you hard. However, the body is very adaptive, and after just a few fasts, it will learn how to access those fat stores to keep you energized, and the side effects are going to fade.

There are a few different problems that a beginner faster may experience. Some of these include:

- Intense hunger: These hunger pains will come and go through the day. These pains are like waves, rather than something that just builds up, so you just need to find ways to distract yourself to make it easier.

- Headaches: These are common when you first start. Take some painkillers to help and drink plenty of fluids.

- Lightheadedness: Some people report feeling a bit lightheaded and spaced out when they go on a fast. When you get to your eating window, eat something a little bit salty.

- Feeling tired: This is going to happen because the body hasn't had time to learn how to access the stores of fat that you have as fuel. A salty drink can help with this.

- Lots of irritability: This can be a big problem when you are near the end of your fast. Planning out the meals that you are going to eat ahead of time can really help. Be aware that your temper may be short, learn how to stay calm or stay away from other people.

- Insomnia: Some people have trouble falling asleep when they go on their first few fasts.

The good news is that most of these are going to fade away within a week or less. Having a good meal plan when you first get started on your intermittent fast and sticking with it, can make a big difference in how well you feel and how successful the fast is. When meal planning, add in lots of nutrients and consider putting one of your bigger meals as the first one to help the body get enough food after going on the fast.

There are also a few things that you can do to reduce the side effects of an intermittent fast and help you be better prepared for this kind of eating plan. First, take it easy for the first few weeks. If you have a big project that is going to occur at work or another stressful situation at hand, then hold off getting started with intermittent fasting.

These situations are going to make you crave food all the time and can already give you headaches and irritability. Adding the intermittent fast on top of that will just make things worse. Consider taking a few days off work if you can or just pick a time that is less stressful and demanding on you to help you get the best results!

Meal planning is another option that you can choose. After you get done with a fast, especially during the first few times, you are going to be really hungry. The body is not used to going such a long time without eating, and as soon as you let it have something, it will want to gobble down as much as it can get ahold of. If you don't have a plan in place, you are going to eat everything in the kitchen and take on way too many calories in the process.

With a good meal plan, you can avoid this issue. You can set up your meals ahead of time, especially for those eating periods right after your fast is ending. That way, when the fast is done, you can just grab the prepared meal and enjoy it, knowing that the meal has all the good nutrients that your body needs and will fill you up.

One thing to remember about meal planning with intermittent fasting is to consider making the first meal after a fast a little bit bigger. Many of us save supper as our biggest meal, but when you are done with a fast, the body is hungry and has been going for a long time without anything to eat. You can certainly provide yourself with a tiny meal after the fast, but you will end up hungry and dissatisfied. A better option is to add a bit more to that first meal to help provide the body with nutrients and to make it feel better. This can make the fast more enjoyable and will ensure you don't go and raid the fridge simply because you are still hungry after your fast.

Chapter 16: Keeping the Fast: What Is Allowed When I Am Fasting?

Many people wonder what they are allowed to eat during their fasted state. They understand that they need to avoid drinks with calories and food and snacks during this time. However, what about some of the items that may not be considered as food, such as gum, breath mints, and even medications? These can provide a type of gray area when it comes to intermittent fasting.

The type of fast that you follow is going to determine what you can have and still maintain for the fast. For example, the regular alternate day fast would have you eat nothing on your fasting days, but the modified version allows you to have up to 500 calories during those fasting days.

On all forms, though, when you are fasting and not eating the one meal allowed, you are required to abstain from food and any drinks that have extra sugars and calories. Let's take a closer look at what is allowed when you are fasting and how to make sure you maintain your fasted state.

The Fasted State

With most forms of an intermittent fast, you will be required to separate your eating and fasting periods. During the eating periods, you are allowed to eat the amount of whole and nutritious foods that the body needs to stay healthy. The more that you can fill up on wholesome foods, the better you will feel when you get to your fasting window again. Focus on whole grains, lean protein, lots of fruits and vegetables, and some healthy dairy products if you can have them. Limit junk and processed food as much as possible.

When you are fasting, though, you need to maintain the fast. You should not eat anything during the fasting portion of this eating program. This allows the body to get into the fat burning state that it needs and can help you to cut down on calories. You can drink as much coffee, tea, and water as you would like to ensure that you stay hydrated.

When it comes to fasting, everything except the liquids that we mentioned before should be avoided. If special circumstances affect you, then you can take that into consideration and make some changes to your fast. But this is an exception and not the rule. For most people who go on an intermittent fast, it is best just to avoid eating anything and only consume the beverages that are listed above to ensure you don't enter dehydration.

If you can put something in your mouth, then it is often going to be considered as something that you should have while you are on your fast. This can include any food and snacks as well as breath mints, gum, and so on. Some fasting protocols may allow for you to consume these products and not consider it as breaking your fast. However, for the most part, it is best to abstain from anything except the non-caloric beverages. Exceptions can be made to things like medication. If you need to take a certain medication each day, you may want to consider following the 5:2 diet or modified alternate fast so that you can take some food in along with your medication to avoid making yourself sick in the process. Supplements and other similar products should be avoided as well until you can eat something with them.

The idea of bulletproof coffee has been introduced recently, and many people wonder if it should be counted as something that breaks the fast. It is coffee, which is one of the beverages allowed during your fast, but this kind of coffee adds in other ingredients that add to your calorie count.

In most instances, you would count it as something that breaks your fast because it does contain other food items and calories as well. You could easily introduce it with the first meal you consume during the day and get the same results. However, if your protocol says that it is not breaking the fast, then it is fine to follow that rule of thumb as well.

The 5:2 Diet and Modified Alternate Fasting

With the modified alternate day fast and the 5:2 diet, there are slightly different rules. These methods do allow you to eat a little bit on your fasting day, but you must keep this to a minimum. You are not allowed to graze on them, and you can't just eat whatever you want, or you will end up back to your original state.

On both versions of intermittent fasting, you can consume up to 500 calories each day. With the 5:2 diet, most people will choose to go with two meals during the day that are 250 calories each. With the modified alternate fasting diet, it is recommended that you eat just one meal, preferably towards the end of the fast or before going to bed, that totals 500 calories. Both can be effective, so you can choose the method that works for you.

When you do eat on both modified versions, you need to make sure that your meals are as nutritious as possible. You will quickly find that eating a bunch of junk is not going to fill you up and can make your fast even more miserable when cravings begin. Think about it.

Two donuts equal 500 calories; however, they are definitely not as filling and nutritious as some turkey or chicken, half a cup of fruit, half a cup of vegetables, and a glass of milk or another similar meal. Choose your meals wisely, and you won't feel as deprived when you are on the fast.

Outside of the 500 calories that you can consume on these modified versions, you need to stick with the same rules as the other fats. You are not allowed to eat anything during the fast. Supplements are often discouraged and should be saved for your eating window to avoid upsetting the stomach. Sodas and other sugary beverages should be avoided, but having water, tea, and coffee is just fine. If you have medications that you must take at certain times, then those are fine, but if you have some freedom in when to take them, wait until your eating window begins again.

Chapter 17: How Do I Track My Progress When I Fast?

When you go on an intermittent fast, you want to see results. But how do you know when you are actually seeing results? Just by looking in the mirror each day, it can be hard to see the results when they happen. Here are a few ways that you can track your progress so that any time you want to check up on yourself, or when you need some extra motivation, you can see how far you have come.

Take Progress Pictures

No one wants to take pictures of themselves when they are at the start of their weight loss journal. However, no matter how uncomfortable it may make you feel to take that picture when you are out of shape, knowing where you are when you get started with fasting, or with any kind of diet plan, can be essential. It is easy for many people just to rely on the scale and let it be the one in charge, but when you consider issues like bodyweight distribution, lean mass gains, and water weight, just looking at the number on the scale can make you miss out on many good changes that are occurring.

Taking the picture is very important. Yes, you do look in the mirror each day already, but since you already do this at least one time a day, the changes that occur are going to be pretty much imperceptible. You need to take the pictures to ensure that you are actually able to see the changes.

Pictures are nice because they give you some separation from the mirror to actually see what is going on. They can allow you to see where you started from and then compare that to where you are now. You can even put the pictures side by side and see if this proves that there are some big changes that have been occurring over time.

When you are getting started on an intermittent fast, make sure that you take pictures of your front, the sides, and the back. Then every few weeks to every month, take these same pictures again. Do not suck in your stomach or push it out; simply stay relaxed and keep the conditions between one picture set to another as similar as you can. This makes it easier to get accurate results and see what is going on. If possible, make sure that you wear the same outfit, take the pictures near the same time of day as each other, and try to stick with the same lighting and angles.

After you have been on your intermittent fast for a few months, take out these pictures and compare them side by side. While you may have been looking into the mirror and not noticing any differences, these pictures should tell a different story. If you followed the intermittent fast the right way and stuck with a healthy diet, you will be able to tell the difference from one picture set to the next, and the difference between the first set of pictures and where you are right now.

Retest the Benchmarks That You Make

This one is often used when it comes to weight lifting, but you can do it with other options as well. Let's look at weightlifting first. When you first get started, take some time to test your strength benchmarks. Check and see how much you can pull and press. What are your squat numbers? This gives you a good idea of your baseline for strength, and then you can figure out which numbers are the most achievable for you to work on. If you ever feel discouraged or like you are not progressing, go back to those benchmark numbers and see how easy they are and how much you can surpass them. You may be surprised at how much stronger you have gotten.

You can do this with any kind of workout. If you were starting to do walking as an exercise, see how fast you can do a mile and then test yourself to see if you could pick up the speed. If you were just starting out and your limit for working out was two miles or 30 minutes of cardio, push it and see how far you can go the next time that you are discouraged.

Make sure that you write these numbers down. They can be great indicators of your current strength, and you can use them to check whether you are getting stronger or not. Many times, we think we are stuck because we aren't able to hit a particularly hard goal. But then we go back and test ourselves, and we find that things really did change; we just didn't notice.

Bring out the Tape Measure

You may be relying on the scale to let you know if you are progressing or not, but it is important to remember that not all the weight you lose is going to be fat. To see if you are actually starting to become leaner and have progressed, even when the scale doesn't seem to want to move, you should bring out a tape measure. Some areas that you can track include your shoulders, biceps, thighs, waist, hips, and chest.

Knowing the measurements around your body could do more than just help you have a physique that is proportionate. Where you store much of your fat can be a big warning sign of complications that are related to obesity. These include things like heart disease, stroke, and diabetes. You can use these measurements to help learn your waist to hip ratio and determine whether you are at a higher risk of these issues as well.

Since intermittent fasting is meant to help you not only lose weight but also lose body fat, the tape measure option is a great idea. Sometimes, the scale is not going to move in the direction that you want it to, and this can be frustrating. However, when you record your measurements on a regular basis, you will see changes in the body, even if the scale is not going the way that you want.

To help you keep track of your own personal measurements, get a journal and write down the date and the measurements for at least your arms, hips, and waist. You can measure any other part of the body that you would like as well to keep you on track. Just hold the tape measure against the skin and measure around, but don't pull it tight or do anything that might give you an inaccurate number.

You should check these measurements on a regular basis. Once a month is a great timeline because it gives you enough time to see some results. If you would like to measure more often or do it every few months, then this is fine as well. Just make sure that you pick out a time limit that is far enough apart, but not too far, so you can actually see your results.

How Much Energy Do You Have Now?

Another benefit that you can get when you go on an intermittent fast is more energy. Once you are done with the first few weeks of your fast, and you can get the body adjusted to this new eating schedule, you are going to see a ton of energy in your daily life. Measuring the amount of energy that you have as you progress on your intermittent fast can help you better track how well the fast is working.

The best way to monitor this is to take a few minutes to journal it. Start a week or so before you decide to go on a fast. Describe how much energy you had, what your mood was like for the day and a few other notes. Then, keep this process up as you start the intermittent fast. Over the next month or so, keep writing. When the time is up, or any time that you want, look back at the notes that you made and see what a difference there is in your mood, energy levels, and outlook on life.

Your Health Markers

Regular visits to the doctor can also help you determine whether you are making progress with your intermittent fast. You can get important tests done, such as a diabetes screening and cholesterol check and then compare the numbers. Many people find that they have more success when they get their doctor on board with them. Before you go on an intermittent fast, consider going in for a checkup with your doctor and getting some easy tests done to see where your numbers are.

After you have been on the fast for six months or so, go back to your doctor and get those numbers checked again. If you were doing a good job staying on your fast and eating healthy foods during your eating window, you are going to be pleasantly surprised by the results that you get when you go back to the doctor.

Measure Your Body Fat

Another way that you can check out whether the intermittent fast is working for you is to measure your body fat. Remember that one of the benefits of going on an intermittent fast is that you get the benefit of losing a lot of belly fat in addition to weight. When you take the time to measure your body fat, you can see just how effective the eating plan is.

Skinfold measurements are a great way to estimate the percentage of fat that is on your body based on the fat that is present underneath the skin. While you may not be happy with the number that you see when you first get started, it is still a good idea to do this measurement because it gives you a place to start when you are dieting.

Keep in mind that sometimes the results can be off by up to six percent. However, if you do the same method each time that you do this, then the percentage loss trend can make it easier to see your progress when it comes to the amount of fat that you lose.

Try on Some Old Clothing

If you are on an intermittent fast and you feel that you have plateaued, or you just want to see how far you have come, then taking out some of your old clothes and trying them on can help you get a good perspective on how far you have come. Sure, you may not have hit the goal that you set, but when you put on a pair of old jeans that used to be tight, and now you are swimming in them, it can certainly make you feel good! While it is a good idea to get rid of many of your old clothes as you get smaller so you don't get tempted to eat bad again and have the clothes there and ready, keeping a few around to use as a measure can be a great way to track your progress.

Use the Scale

Another way that you can measure and track the amount of progress that you make while intermittent fasting is to use the scale. This helps you to see exactly how much weight you have lost and how far you have gone since you first got started. The reason that it is so far down on the list is that it isn't always the best indicator.

Sure, you do want to see your weight go down. This helps you to fight off many health conditions and shows that you are healthier and more fit overall. But if you are adding in exercise, especially strength training, you may find that the numbers don't always add up the right way. Muscle weighs more than fat so while you are burning fat with your fast, you may be building up muscle, and that can give you a higher number on the scale. Use the scale as a tool, but make sure that it is used as a complement to the other methods we discuss here.

Chapter 18: Should I Add Any Exercise into My Fast?

The most effective intermittent fast is one where you add lots of healthy exercises as well. Intermittent fasting can do a great deal of good when it comes to cutting calories and helping you lose weight, but the other part of the equation is for you to add in some exercise as well. Exercise can help you maintain your muscle mass, burn more calories than fasting alone and give you more energy to get through the day.

A common question that people on an intermittent fast may have is how they can add in more exercise to their day and which exercises are the best. To keep it simple, any exercise that you enjoy doing and that you will keep doing for the long term is going to be perfect. However, there are times when a specific workout will be more effective or enjoyable to you.

If you can, it is best to do a good mixture of workouts with some weight training, cardio, and strength training mixed together. But doing one type of exercise that you love is better than not doing anything at all. Let's explore some of the different types of workouts that you can consider with intermittent fasting, and how to do them safely to get the best results.

Weight Lifting and Intermittent Fasting

When it comes to intermittent fasting, many people like to begin a weight lifting or strength training workout. This can be beneficial in several ways. First, it helps you to build up lots of lean and strong muscles that make you look trimmer and can burn through more fat and calories than just intermittent fasting alone. Strength training can also work when you are in a fasted state because you don't need to burn up fuel as quickly as you do with cardio.

Many people who add weight training to their routine will do it while they are in their fasted state, although it is fine to add in anywhere you have time. Doing this during the fasted state can help you burn through even more glycogen than before, giving you better results.

If you do choose to weight train during a fast, try to set it up so that you end your fasting window right after the exercise is done. This way, you can get the benefits of training while fasted, but then you can provide the body with the nutrients it needs to repair those muscles once the workout is done.

With weight training and intermittent fasting, fewer reps with more weight are the best option. This helps you to get the stronger muscle that looks lean, without having to spend hours in the gym. Start out small, and perhaps even skip the workouts in the beginning. You will get stronger and will be able to take on more weight but remember that this is a time when your body is adjusting, and you never want to overdo it.

Is HIIT a Good Idea to Add into My Exercise Plan

One thing that you may want to consider adding into your exercise program is HIIT or high-intensity interval training. This type of exercise can really help add in many extra health benefits, and it doesn't require you spending hours in the gym like other methods.

Researchers have taken time to look at HIIT exercises and found that they can be effective. It has been shown that doing three rounds of 20 seconds of HIIT three times a week can give the body as many benefits as you get while running on the treadmill. Instead of spending all that time running on the treadmill or at the gym, you could spend about ten to 15 minutes on your workout and get the same benefits.

For those who are just getting started on their own intermittent fast and aren't used to the effects, or those who aren't used to doing a lot of working out, it can be great news to help them get started. You will get a ton of benefits with just a short burst of exercise, and who wouldn't want to see that?

You get some choices when it comes to HIIT. You can either make the whole workout based on this idea or find ways to add it into your regular workout. For example, you can either do ten minutes of the spurts or go out for a two-mile walk and add in three or four rounds with a sprint that lasts about 20 seconds each. Both will provide you with good benefits to your health in a shorter amount of time.

Do I Need to Worry About Preserving My Muscles During an Intermittent Fast?

Many experts agree that out of the health benefits that you get out of exercise and diet, 80 percent comes from your diet. The other 20 percent will come from the exercise that you do. This means that it is more important to concentrate on consuming the right kinds of foods to help you lose weight and keep your muscle strength intact. However, adding exercise to the mixture can really help you get healthier as well.

Some research looked at the data of participants who were on the show *The Biggest Loser*. The information that was looked at for this research included the resting metabolic rate, the total amount of energy used, and the total body fat of all the participants and these numbers were measured three times. They were measured right when the program began, after six weeks into the program, and then finally done after 30 weeks.

Researchers found that the diet the participants consumed was the most responsible for the weight that they lost. And only about 65 percent of that loss in weight came from body fat. The rest came from a loss in lean muscle mass. Exercise alone resulted in an only fat loss with a slight increase in lean muscle mass. This means that it is possible to lose a little bit of muscle mass with just diet alone but adding in exercise will ensure that you can maintain and even grow that muscle mass while eating a healthy diet like on an intermittent fast.

Chapter 19: What If I'm Not Seeing Results from My Fast?

An intermittent fast is a great way for you to get in the best health of your life and lose weight all at the same time. However, there are times when you may not be seeing the exact results that you want. When this happens, many fasters ask why they aren't losing weight. There is usually a pretty simple explanation for this. The most common one is that you have lost some weight, but because of increased muscle tone, or the natural variations that occur in the weight of your body through the day, it isn't showing up on the scale. There are several reasons why you may not be seeing the results of your intermittent fast right away, and some of these are:

- *How long have you been on the intermittent fast?*

The amount of time that you have been on the intermittent fast can make a difference. If you just got started with fasting, you are not going to see a ton of weight loss in just a week. It will take a bit of time for your body to adapt to this new eating plan. While many people who go on a fast see results in weight loss right away, this early loss can often be because there are changes in the amount of water the body holds onto.

This means that one of the reasons that you don't see much weight loss is because you didn't lose a lot of water in the beginning. Even using a tape measure to check your waist and other parts of the body, it may be a little bit slow to show the differences that are occurring based on where you lose the fat.

If you have been on the fast for a long time and you have stopped losing weight, or it seems like you are hitting a plateau, several things could be to blame here. These can include:

oIf you are having weight loss, but it is slow, the actual weight that is lost can be hidden by many other natural variations that we go through each day. Our weight can vary by about two pounds up or down due to the way that the body holds onto water or the foods that are passing through our system. If you were losing weight and then it seems to stop, it could be because of some of the variations that happen in your body. You may be holding onto water more or even gaining some muscle.

oSecond, as you start to lose weight, the body is going to need less energy to survive, so the speed of weight loss is going to slow down, and it may even plateau. To help make more progress, you will need to make efforts to use more energy each day by increasing your levels of activity. Combine this with a reduction in the number of calories that you take in each day. Any time that you stall in your weight loss, consider recalculating your daily energy needs to see if you need to change it up.

oThird, as you get comfortable with the intermittent fast, it is sometimes easy to let things slip a little, and you may not be as strict about your calorie intake on the fasting days or the length of your fast. This loss of focus can be a reason that you are not losing weight any longer or a reason why you have stalled out.

If any of these are true with you, it is important just to keep calm and wait it out for a bit. You may need to wait a few weeks to find out if you really plateaued or not. In the meantime, recalculate the energy that you expend during the day and check that you are not eating more calories or cutting into your fast earlier than you think. If nothing is working, it may be time to upgrade to a different version of the fast, such as going from the 5:2 diet to the alternate day fast.

• *How much and how quickly do you want to lose weight?*

If you are at a pretty healthy weight and you don't need to lose much, then you will find that the rate at which you lose weight is going to be a lot slower compared to someone who has quite a bit to lose. If you are already close to your healthy weight range and you are in shape, and you are trying to lose a few pounds in just a week or two, then you may end up being disappointed in this process. Intermittent fasting can still work, but you must realize that it is going to take more time for those who are closer to their ideal and healthy weight range.

As you start to carry around less fat, your body is going to slow the weight loss through several different methods. Although scientists are still in debate about whether our bodies have a preferred set weight at which weight loss efforts are going to stall, in practice, many people have this problem. If you are already at a pretty healthy weight for you, then it may be time to consider whether you need to make some revisions to your target when it comes to weight loss.

If you still want to lose some weight, or you have a lot of weight to lose, and you get stalled, then it is possible that some medical issues are the reason behind this struggle. Some conditions like fibromyalgia, PCOS, and thyroid problems can all make it difficult for you to lose the weight that you would like.

The best thing that you can do is think about the amount that you need to lose to help make yourself healthier rather than giving yourself a target that is hard to reach. You also need to accept that weight loss can be a very slow process since intermittent fasting is all about changing your lifestyle for the better. Intermittent fasting is not just a fad that you try for a few weeks; it is something that you stick with for the long haul, even if that means you don't lose weight as quickly as you want.

Since this type of eating is more about sticking to it for the long term, it may be time to consider whether a change to your method of fasting is the way that would help you lose weight quicker. Changing things up on occasion can keep you from getting bored with your version of intermittent fasting and could help to shorten your eating window, so it is easier to lose weight. Why not try out the alternate day fast for a few weeks or change up your eating, so you take in fewer carbs? These simple changes to the fast can make a big difference in how much you enjoy the fast and even the amount that you can lose.

- *Are you eating too much during your eating window or eating the wrong types of foods?*

Another reason why you may not be losing weight is that you are overeating during your non-fasting times. While intermittent fasting can help you to reduce your caloric intake, it is not a cure-all, and it is still possible for an individual to eat too much during their non-fasting periods.

The first thing to consider, if you lost a lot of weight, is that you might need to take in even less food to sustain your body. If it's been a while since you went through and figured out how many calories you need to consume, then now is the time to do it again. You may find that you are inadvertently taking in more calories than your body needs, and it is time to cut it down a little bit more.

In some cases, you may be doing well on a fast, and then suddenly, the days when you are super hungry start to happen more frequently. Intermittent fasting can help to control the appetite, but sometimes, those extra hungry days are going to start getting out of hand. When this happens, it may be time to add in an extra fast day to your schedule, or at least extending the length of your fasting period to help get that appetite back under control.

If you are suffering from insulin resistance, be aware that your body is going to be very sensitive to any carbs that you take in, especially refined carbs and sugars. Carbs are going to stimulate the body to release insulin, which makes it hard for you to burn any of your stored fat. And for some people, once they take in a few carbs, they get into a cycle of being hungry and having a lot of cravings at the same time.

If this sounds like something that happens to you, it may be time to consider changing the type of diet you are on. Most people are just fine sticking with a diet that allows some whole grains and other carbs, but for those who are sensitive to them and who seem to have trouble on their fast, it may be time to go on a low carb diet. With this kind of diet, you will avoid all carbs on your fast days and then severely reduce carbs on your non-fasting times. This may seem extreme, but you will be amazed at how much it can help when you are struggling with keeping your calories in check with an intermittent fast.

Before we end, a word about alcohol while fasting. Some people find that drinking alcohol can slow down the amount of weight they can lose while also increasing their appetite on those non-fast days. This substance can also make it hard on fasting days. This is because alcohol is going to influence how the body can handle carbs, and this particularly affects the liver. If you do drink while you are fasting, it may be time to consider cutting down on how much alcohol you consume. You don't have to give it up completely but be careful and make sure that you reduce or eliminate it the day before one of your fasts to get the best results.

Intermittent fasting can be a fun way to help you lose weight and get in the best shape of your life. However, there are also times when you will hit a plateau and can't seem to lose any more weight, despite following all the same steps that you did in the past. When this happens to you, it can be really frustrating, and you want to figure out how to make it change. Follow some of the tips that are in this chapter, and it won't be long before your weight loss begins to happen again!

Conclusion

Thanks for making it through to the end of *Intermittent Fasting: How to Lose Weight, Burn Fat, and Increase Mental Clarity without Having to Give up All Your Favorite Foods*. It should have been informative and provided you with all the tools needed to achieve your goals whatever they may be.

The next step is to decide if intermittent fasting is the right eating protocol for you to follow. This eating plan will provide you with a ton of great benefits and can easily help you lose weight while not feeling deprived in the process. And with the different methods that are available with intermittent fasting, it is something you will really enjoy and can easily fit into your daily schedule without much hassle.

Inside this guidebook, we looked at an intermittent fast and how it can be so much more effective than your current eating plan. With the current American diet, we are taking in too many calories and getting into a horrible cycle that makes us sick. The body may crave those bad foods because they provide it with an easy and constant source of fuel, but we are slowly setting ourselves up for a whole bunch of chronic illnesses.

Intermittent fasting helps us to change all that. It allows us the option to cut down on how many calories we consume during the day while also naturally speeding up the metabolism. Add in there that you will not give the body a constant source of glucose any longer, so it must rely on stored glycogen and other resources. It is no wonder that intermittent fasting can help solve health problems while also helping us lose weight.

We also looked at some of the basics that come with intermittent fasting, how to get started, the different health benefits you can get from fasting, the steps that you can follow to get the most out of this fasting method, the side effects that you may notice when you first get started, the things that you can do if fasting doesn't seem to be working right for you and how to fix these issues, and so much more.

While there may be many different eating and diet plans out there, intermittent fasting is one that seems to work well for so many people. It helps them learn how to listen to their body, how to eat more healthily, and how to allow their body to get into fat burning mode all on its own.

Finally, if you found this book useful in any way, a review on Amazon is always appreciated!

CPSIA information can be obtained
at www.ICGtesting.com
Printed in the USA
LVHW080916291220
675316LV00004B/25

9 781647 482855